P9-CCO-957

A Series of Catastrophes & Miracles

A Series of Catastrophes & Miracles

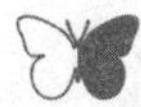

A True Story of Love, Science, and Cancer

MARY ELIZABETH WILLIAMS

NATIONAL GEOGRAPHIC

Washington, D.C.

Published by National Geographic Partners, LLC

Library of Congress Cataloging-in-Publication Data
Names: Williams, Mary Elizabeth, (Journalist), author.
Title: A series of catastrophes and miracles : a true story of love, science, and cancer / Mary Elizabeth Williams.
Description: Washington, D.C. : National Geographic, [2016]
Identifiers: LCCN 2015033584 | ISBN 9781426216336 (hardback)
Subjects: LCSH: Williams, Mary Elizabeth, (Journalist),--Health. | Metastasis. | Cancer--Patients--Biography. | Cancer in women--Patients--Biography. | Women--Health and hygiene. | BISAC: BIOGRAPHY & AUTOBIOGRAPHY / Personal Memoirs. | BIOGRAPHY & AUTOBIOGRAPHY / Women. | HEALTH & FITNESS / Diseases / Cancer.
Classification: LCC RC269.5 .W55 2016 | DDC 362.19699/40092--dc23
LC record available at http://lccn.loc.gov/2015033584

Since 1888, the National Geographic Society has funded more than 12,000 research, exploration, and preservation projects around the world. National Geographic Partners distributes a portion of the funds it receives from your purchase to National Geographic Society to support programs including the conservation of animals and their habitats.

National Geographic Partners, LLC
1145 17th Street NW
Washington, DC 20036-4688 USA

Become a member of National Geographic and activate your benefits today at natgeo.com/jointoday.

For information about special discounts for bulk purchases, please contact National Geographic Books Special Sales: ngspecsales@ngs.org

For rights or permissions inquiries, please contact National Geographic Books Subsidiary Rights: ngbookrights@ngs.org

Interior design: Melissa Farris

Printed in the United States of America

16/QGF-RRDML/1

For Debbie

Author's Note

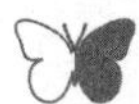

This is a work of nonfiction. I have tried throughout to present scientific facts and history as accurately as possible and to the best of my ability—albeit as someone with a decidedly unscientific background.

For the narrative aspects, I have relied heavily on the notes, date books, and journals I kept, my medical records, and the stories I published throughout the experience. I've also depended on the very generous cooperation of many of the individuals who were present for and participated in the events depicted. I am exceedingly grateful to them for letting me interview them, for giving me access to their own journals and personal stories, and for helping me reconstruct many scenes and conversations.

There are no composite characters here. Everyone within has a real-life counterpart. I have, however, changed names and identifying details of certain individuals to protect their privacy. I have also in a few instances condensed conversations and events—mostly involving doctor visits—that took place over more than one episode into single scenes for the sake of clarity.

There is no doubt that everyone involved in this tale has his or her version of how it all went down. This is mine.

Portions of this story have appeared, in slightly different format, in Salon and in the *New York Times*.

SPOILER:
I lived.

CHAPTER 1

Cancer Club Night

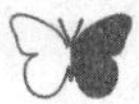

January 10, 2012

It's a bad time for the phone to ring. Jeff is already down the hall at his caregiver group; Lucy and Bea are downstairs doing arts and crafts with the other kids in Noogieland. My own support group is just about to start, and our facilitator Marlena is strict that outside interruptions—and latecomers—are not tolerated. I glance at the phone and see that the call is from an unfamiliar number. Do I answer it and risk banishment, or spend the next two hours going crazy wondering who it was from—especially today, of all days?

The family started coming to Gilda's Club in the fall—right after the rediagnosis—and since then we've grown to treasure our Tuesday nights here. It's a weekly source of stability and support in the chaos of my cancer. We love the unexpected community that my disease has provided us, and the raucous laughter we always wind up sharing within these walls. We love the friends who've become family over the past few months. But sometimes this little clubhouse is a hard place to be. Eventually, everybody leaves it—and there are only a few ways out. The hoped-for option is by getting better.

I have a lot to talk about tonight. This morning, I had examined my shampoo bottle as I washed my hair and wondered if I would make it to the bottom of it. Lately I weigh the practicality of renewing my *New Yorker* subscription, and the uncertainty of making plans for summer vacation when it's only early January. I wonder if I will finish a canister of oatmeal, or if my bottle of Tabasco will outlast my presence in this world. These are the things I think about these days, because I have Stage 4 melanoma—a condition that typically grants people like me only a miserly handful of months to live. These are the things I had contemplated today before going for my first set of scans since starting my clinical trial. The ones that will tell me if the tumors in my lung and soft tissue are shrinking, or if I'm closer to dying the painful, merciless death of late-stage cancer.

I am now three months into the trial. Tomorrow is my children's shared birthday. Lucy will be twelve and Bea will be eight. They're so in sync, they even came into the world on the same date, four years apart. Whatever else happens next, we will mark another milestone. We will celebrate another year.

I have my next treatment in two days. The side effects haven't been too debilitating—the word I keep using is "tolerable." I'm exhausted all the time, have an itchy rash, get dizzy spells, and my sense of taste is off. But I get to keep what's left of my hair and not throw up, so who's complaining? Especially when the tumor on my back—the tender purple lump that rests right under my bra strap—has been looking smaller since the first treatment. Dr. Wolchok says it's very encouraging, though I'm trying not to get my hopes up. People with multiple distant metastases don't usually get happy endings. We usually just get endings. We get doctors asking us if we're in pain, an unspoken "yet" dangling from their lips. We get the understanding that the cancer could be dancing anywhere in our bodies, eating our organs.

Earlier today, I had guzzled down a jug of disgusting orange fluid and I'd held my breath as technicians took pictures of my insides, wondering what they would reveal about the monster within me. "Whatever happens," I'd told Jeff when I called him afterward, "I can probably try to talk them into operating on my lung." I wasn't sure I believed it. The lung tumor is in a delicate place, and if my condition is worsening, my options are diminishing.

Thank God Debbie has been doing okay. She's been on Abraxane since September, and this round of chemo seems to be going well, even if the fuzzy new Chia Pet growth of hair she'd finally grown back over the summer is gone once again. "I have one eyelash left," she'd told me the last time I called. "It's driving me crazy." She doesn't know how long her course will be this time. The doctors keep saying they have to wait and see how she's doing, how her CA 125 numbers are.

Debbie is tired of the constant rigors of getting her parking validated at the hospital parking lot. She's irritated with her chemo port, and she's over this whole having poisons flowing through her body thing. She's also scared of what happens when the chemo ends.

I'm scared too, but I feel like I could live through anything else they dole out on the fourth floor of Memorial Sloan Kettering if they can just get me to the spring. Just to see the cherry blossoms one more time. But even if my tests today tell me that the cancer has been arrested, there's still the nagging doubt, the skepticism that comes when you've already had one recurrence. If I live through the next few months, what will become of me when the initial course of treatment is scheduled to end? How many reprieves will I get in this life? Tonight, I'll settle for one. Tonight, that's what I want to talk about with my group.

So when the unknown number appears on my iPhone right now, I am sorely tempted to ignore it. But I pick it up anyway, just in case it's important, as I scurry guiltily out of the room toward the hall.

The voice on the other end is Dr. Wolchok's. "I have your results," he says. He must be calling from his own phone instead of his usual office one. Dammit. If it weren't grave, he'd wait till my appointment this Thursday. He wouldn't be calling me from his own phone at night.

"Hey, how's it going?" I ask, like this is a social call and I give a damn how he's doing this evening.

He wastes no time. "I'm calling because I have good news," he replies. "I would have contacted you earlier, but I didn't want to tease you until we had confirmation on everything from the lab. We got your scans, and the tumor on your back has completely receded. The one in your lung is gone."

I leave my body for a moment as the universe abruptly lurches in an entirely new direction. "Did you say gone?" I ask. Then I add, because I want to be sure I understand what he's saying, "Now, what does that mean, exactly?"

"Gone," he repeats. "Your tumors are completely gone. You present no evidence of disease. So we'll see you again on Thursday and we'll run your blah blah blah and you'll come back blah blah blah."

I don't comprehend him. His voice has become the droning horn of a grown-up in a Charlie Brown special. I'm too busy simultaneously registering shock and crying. As he continues, I sleepwalk into Jeff's meeting room. I simply point at him and beckon him out. He follows obediently as I say, "Thank you, Doctor," and hang up.

Jeff regards my tearstained face with apprehension. "He says it's all gone," I say. He looks utterly bewildered for a moment, at the blubbering woman giving him impossibly happy news. Then a smile spreads across his face. He holds up his hand for a high five that melts into a hug. "Okay," he says, his eyes damp. "Okay, I'll take it." We don't jump up and down and whoop like contestants on a game show; it's too unreal. Instead, he goes back into his room and I quickly scoot into mine. My metastatic, eager-to-kill-me cancer is gone. In just three months. Three months and a hundred years of research and my doctor's entire life's work.

Everyone else is already well settled in when I return to our group. Cassandra is curled up in her usual spot on the couch like a sleepy cat. As soon as I stagger, red-faced, into the room, she shoots me a worried look, and flashes her thumb—first up, and then down—in silent question. I reply with a hasty thumbs-up as I grab my seat next to her, and she squeezes my hand reassuringly.

Tonight is the last time I will ever see Cassandra. She will be dead in a month. Her sons, who are currently downstairs screaming circles around the girls, will be the next to leave the children's family group and go into the children's bereavement group. Tonight, though, she and I sit hand in hand on the couch, friends who, in other circumstances, might have met and bonded over playground parties and homework hassles and passionate debates over where to get the best hot chocolate in town. Now instead fighting tooth and nail not to leave their children.

Marlena breaks the spell. "If everybody's here, I guess we can start," she says. "Who would like to go first tonight?"

I raise my hand. As Cassandra gives me an encouraging nod, I say, "I would."

CHAPTER 2

Best Summer Ever

August 11, 2010

The thing that tried to take my life was as big as the eraser on a no. 2 pencil. Significantly smaller than a bullet. Less formidable looking than a drop of poison. I can't remember the first time I noticed it, because there wasn't much to notice. I only know that it was sometime in early summer, and that as the season slipped from the bright cool of June to the muggy stillness of August, I realized that the scab on my scalp was still there, and the fact that it wasn't healing was getting old.

I felt it when I washed my hair, and wondered what I'd managed to do to myself this time. I'm always discovering some new nick or bruise or scratch or gaping wound I hadn't perceived at the time it was inflicted, usually in the course of chasing after the kids. It wasn't causing me pain; it didn't itch or ooze. It was such a minor nuisance, such a superficial imperfection that my hair covered anyway, that it hardly seemed worth a call to the skin doctor. But I didn't want this stupid bump on my head indefinitely either, and figured some ointment or antibiotics never hurt anybody.

When I went to see her last week, my dermatologist hadn't offered any pills or topical solutions, though. Instead, she'd knit her eyebrows together and meaningfully sucked in the air between her teeth. "That looks like skin cancer," she'd said. "I'm going to need to biopsy it."

Even then, I figured it was no big deal. I know lots of people who've had basal cell carcinomas removed. It's the sort of thing people call "the good kind of cancer." A little scrape. A little Band-Aid. A little scar. Lucky for me, mine was in a place nobody would even see. I felt something pinch the top of my head, and the doctor said she'd get back to me in a few days.

It's 10:15 on a Wednesday morning when I get the call.

The kids are downtown in Chelsea at their summer day camp. Jeff is at his office in the West Village, writing copy. And I am working at home, draining the last of my morning coffee and plugging away on a story about a belligerent McDonald's patron whose temper tantrum has gone viral, when the trill of the phone disrupts my train of thought.

I've had calls from doctors before, even a few unnerving ones that included phrases like "more tests" and "procedure." Right away, though, this one is different. It cuts right to the chase. No chitchat or "How are you today?" Not this time.

"Hi, Mary Elizabeth. It's Dr. Silver," the voice says. "We got your biopsies back, and I'm sorry to tell you this, but you have malignant melanoma."

This is how the bottom drops out of your world, in ten seconds. It's the sound of your doctor telling you, "I'm sorry."

To her credit, she truly does sound sorry. My pretty dermatologist, the lady with the twins in kindergarten and the cute shoes, feels a pity for me I don't yet even comprehend. "I've made an appointment for you with my colleague. You're going to go to Sloan Kettering tomorrow," she continues. It's 10:16.

That's when the first sickening wave of reality hits. Sloan Kettering. The cancer place. She wants me there tomorrow. Dr. Silver is speaking much too quickly now, and my hands are groping for pen and paper and my brain is flailing to grasp her words. "Because of the size and the depth of the melanoma, they're likely going to have to be aggressive in treating it. The doctor will probably talk to you about surgery and some form of adjuvant treatment like chemo or radiation. You may also need some further therapy for your immune system. They'll be able to discuss your treatment course once they determine how much it's spread." *How much it's spread.*

"It's a lot of information, and I'm sure you have a lot of questions," she says. I do. How am I going to finish writing my story? What am I going to tell my children? What do you mean, malignant? I'm frantically scribbling notes as she speaks, grabbing on to one word in fifty. Aggressive. Adjuvant. Lymph nodes. Immune. I don't understand. So instead, I just dully say, "Thank you. I guess we'll be speaking again soon."

My desk looks the same. My nearly finished story is still on the computer screen in front of me. And I have cancer.

Thomas, my editor at Salon, is expecting a story filed in ten minutes. Thomas doesn't know. Nobody who isn't a doctor knows. *I have a secret,* I think. Five days ago, I wrote a feature in Salon about Christopher Hitchens and his cancer diagnosis. Five days from now, *The Big C,* Showtime's heavily promoted new series about a kooky, fair-skinned mom with life-threatening melanoma, is premiering, and I'd been planning on writing about that. My timing is hilarious. "I'm running late," I tell him in IM.

A clipped reply boings back, "How late?" I can feel the flash of impatience from the other side of the screen.

I look at his words but I don't reply right away, because I don't want to say it. When I say it, it will be real and everything will be different. Except it already is real. It already has happened.

"Dude," I reply. "I have cancer."

"Oh God," he writes back, "I'm so sorry." Because he doesn't know what else to do, he adds, "Take your time." And because I don't know what else to do either, I get back to work and file my story.

Thank God for the raw, motivating power of shock. It's what gets us out of burning buildings. It's what guides us calmly to the emergency room when the hospital calls to say a loved one has just been brought in. It's what finishes stories when we're on deadline.

Next, I write an email to my editors. It reads, "Just learned I have malignant cancer. Taking rest of day off. Going to Sloan Kettering tomorrow and back online Friday." I hit send. Then, and only then, do I put my head in my hands and cry.

When I've composed myself enough to speak, I call Jeff at his job. Jeff and I—well, it's complicated. We met and married in our 20s. In the ensuing two decades, we lived in three cities and seven apartments and had two kids and more jobs than I can count, and then, like a lot of other couples in this world, we broke up. We separated more than two years ago. And until just a few minutes ago, I'd have said that our marital crisis was the hardest thing that I'd ever gone through.

But even in the worst moments of our estrangement—and the breakup of a long marriage is no picnic—we held ourselves to two strict rules: We would always put our daughters Lucy and Bea first, and we would always try to treat each other with respect. To that end, we showed up together for every school play, every teacher conference, and every birthday party. We even rented an apartment right downstairs from our co-op, so the girls would never be far from both parents. If we'd never had the kids, we would have evaporated from each other's lives. Instead, with all that togetherness, I suppose it was inevitable we'd fall for each other eventually.

Our new relationship ignited as slowly as the marriage had died, and in much the same manner. Old feelings subsided, and in time found themselves replaced with different ones. That's life for you.

Things change, and then they keep right on changing. After the initial pain of the breakup diminished, we'd formed a deep and satisfying friendship. Then one day a few months ago he'd cracked a joke, and I'd laughed, and he'd said, with a sexy new confidence, "In case you hadn't noticed, I'm flirting with you." It felt good to be flirted with. It felt good to flirt back. We'd gone on a date—one that had led to more. The past spring and summer had been a monumental leap of faith for both of us, and a damn fun one at that. I had always hoped that after my marriage ended, I'd someday be able to give my heart away again. Sure enough, this had been the year I had fallen in love. It just happened to be with the father of my children.

We both still find ourselves at a loss when friends ask if we're "back together." The phrase implies retreat, whereas we have been happily regarding this as a very different chapter. It's not the starry romance that happens when you're young; and unlike last time, it hasn't hinged upon guarantees. We now both understand that life can't always pan out exactly as you'd imagined. "Let's just take it one day at a time," he'd said recently, a notion I'd found, at this stage in life, far more solid and real than the naively ironclad vows we'd so confidently exchanged so long ago. Now I have to tell this poor bastard that the woman he chose—twice—is massively, medically defective. You want to take it one day at a time? Well, let's see how you take this day, buddy. Because it's a whopper.

"Hey, honey, what's up?" he asks cheerfully, surprised by my late–mid-morning interruption.

"I just got off the phone with Dr. Silver," I blurt back in a breathless stream, "and I have melanoma and it sounds like it's bad and I have to go to Sloan Kettering tomorrow."

He doesn't answer at once. My words tumbled out so quickly they need some time, like the light from a distant star, to reach him. "Okay," he says finally, slowly. "I did not expect this. I did not expect you to say you have malignant cancer."

"Neither did I," I say.

"Obviously, I'm going with you tomorrow," he quickly adds. "We'll get more information and we'll find out what we need to do and then we'll do it. You know, my uncle Jim had melanoma or skin cancer, one of those, and it wasn't so bad."

"Right," I say. "Right. And if it is bad, I'll probably have great access to wigs and weed, so that's a plus."

I wish I wasn't alone in this apartment right now, so I wouldn't have to freak out all by myself. I'm glad I'm alone, so I can freak out in uninterrupted solitude. Imagine if I'd been in an office cubicle or waiting for the Bx20 bus to Marble Hill when I got this life-changing news.

"Is there anything you need?" he asks.

"Just to hear it'll be okay," I answer.

This time, there's only the slightest pause. It's the sort of change in the rhythm of speech that only two people who've known each other for ages can even perceive, that microbeat before speaking. "Of course it will," he says, and I want so badly to believe he's telling the truth.

Throughout the summer, as my scab refused to diminish on its own, I'd typed my way through my share of meaningless search terms, never once getting near an inkling of what was really going on in my body. "Infected cut." "Bug bite." "Hair dye allergic reaction." Nothing of any use, nothing that prepared me. So now let's try a new one: "Malignant melanoma scalp."

Oh, dear. Dr. Google is definitely not your friend. Melanoma is one of the most diagnosed forms of cancer among younger people, and over the past 30 years, its incidence rate has been skyrocketing. But it doesn't always have to be a big life-or-death deal. Even though it unsurprisingly accounts for "the large majority of skin cancer deaths," the American Society of Clinical Oncology notes that its overall five-year survival rate is 91 percent. Unfortunately, it turns out my kind is different. As I search, up pops a *New York Times* story and a quote: "Research finds that having a first invasive melanoma on the scalp or neck leads to twice the risk of dying in five to ten years as having it on the extremities, trunk, face, or ears." An April 2008 report out of the University of North Carolina warns, "Scalp/neck location is associated with poorer melanoma survival."

That's inspiration enough to then detour right toward the most messed-up path I can think of: my diagnosis combined with the phrase "survival rate." Melanoma is usually very responsive to treatment when caught early. But right now in 2010, when it's diagnosed later, the phrase "less than 10 percent" comes up in a heartbeat next to "ten-year survival." I guess this isn't the good kind of cancer.

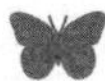

My daughters are only ten and six years old. For the first of what will be a thousand times, a thought occurs to me: If I died now, for the rest of their lives, people would ask them, how old were you when you lost your mom? How much of her do you remember? They would feel sorry for them, the two sisters without a mother. I look down at my hands, and realize they're shaking. I push my chair away from my desk and walk into the bedroom, where I sit down on the edge of the bed and stare blankly at the apartment buildings across our narrow uptown Manhattan street. This beautiful day. This perfect morning. This catastrophe.

I stay frozen on the bed for I don't know how long, until I decide at last that I need to get the hell out of the apartment. I put on my big, cheap, Jackie O–size sunglasses from Target, slather on a thick layer of sunscreen as if my life depended on it, and head out the door, blindly moving forward. As I walk toward the A train, I feel the heat of the August sun on my head and instinctively reach my hand to my hair. It's warm to the touch, igniting the cancer cells in my skin beneath it, no doubt. I feel defenseless and exposed.

It's not as if my vampire-grade, chalk white complexion has escaped my attention until now. I am in every way a textbook candidate for melanoma. Incredibly pale and freckly? Check. Had one blistering sunburn—or more—before age 18? Check. What about that bonus childhood head injury on the Log Flume at Six Flags Great Adventure, the one that left me with the tiniest patch of scarred, hairless skin right at the crown of my head? Just big enough for the sun to do its work. Yet I've lingered in the shade my whole life, a barrier of SPF 35 and a touch of Jergens Natural Glow perpetually standing between the world and me. It just never once, in all my years, crossed my mind how much I needed to protect my head. I thought that was what the hair was for. Oh lordy, Nicole Kidman was right. We gingers should always be wearing a hat.

It's a straight shot on the train from our neighborhood at the tip of Manhattan to Columbus Circle, and from there I walk directly toward Lincoln Center. Just last week I took the girls for Chinese food at Ollie's, right up the street, and afterward we ate ice cream from the Mister Softee truck. It was sublime. On Saturday, I had been swinging 25 feet above the ground in a trapeze class on Governors Island. Yesterday, my Facebook status was "Best summer ever." Now, abruptly, it's become the worst. It's become, maybe, the last.

Then I think, No. Not yet. As I approach the fountain, I fish a piece of change out of my purse. The copper glints in the afternoon sun as I hold it tightly for the length of time it takes to make a wish, and then fling it toward the water, where it lands with a small splash. I put on my sunglasses and walk away, back toward the subway, with tears streaming down my face.

Later, I am stumbling through the motions of making dinner when Jeff walks in with the girls, worn out from their respective days at work and camp. "Mommmeeeeeeee!" the kids squeal. I throw my arms around them like I haven't seen them in a year, inhaling deeply the smell of their skin and the sunshine in their hair.

"How are you doing?" Jeff asks. I look up at him, and my red-rimmed eyes are answer enough. We whisper briefly in the kitchen on the topics of hospital appointments, subway logistics, and paralyzing fear as I drain spaghetti.

Over plates of pasta, I try to tell the girls. But the thing about children is that they tend to not sit primly around the dinner table, waiting for grown-ups to tell them about their cancer. Mine have spent the day at Rye Playland, so they're especially cranked up with tales of nausea-courting thrill rides and funnel cake abuse. Lucy and Bea are racing to tell me about who forgot her lunch box on the bus and who screamed loudest on the Ferris wheel, clamoring for more garlic bread and another glass of milk. I can barely get a word in edgewise, and anyway, I have nothing planned for when I do. No inspirational, Churchill-like speech about how we shall fight this on the beaches and the landing grounds. Instead, I just look at their happy, exhausted faces one last time before their lives are going to change in ways I can't even fathom, this final moment before we become Cancer Family. *Remember this,* I think. Remember what it felt like before it all changed. Then I say, "I have something to tell you about my day too.

"I got a call from the doctor," I continue, "and you know that little bump I had looked at last week? Well, we found out that it's cancer. So Mama is going to meet a new doctor tomorrow, and she's going to have an operation, and she might have to have some treatment that could make her seem sick. You know, like Grandpa." Then I exhale.

They don't really know what cancer is. They know that Grandpa had an operation last year and that they went to visit him in the hospital. They know that the gift shop was very pretty. They know that he did something called chemo and that he was okay for a few months but now he has to do chemo again and get a weird button stuck under his skin, near the collarbone. They don't have a lifetime of dread associated with the word.

Bea—sweet, cheerful, sunny Bea—looks over at her big sister to gauge how she should react. And it's not from my words but the look on Lucy's face that she realizes it's serious. She widens her eyes dramatically. "Oh no!" she says. "You have to have yucky medicine?"

I smile. "Maybe."

"Because you have cancer," she continues. "Even if you don't look sick." Then another thought occurs to her. "So are you going to get better or are you going to die?" she asks curiously. Six-year-olds—not famed for their subtlety.

That's where Lucy, my wise, sardonic big girl of few words, steps in. "She's going to get better," she declares. "Right?"

I look across the table and straight into her somber brown eyes. She's a clever, funny girl, but her default mode is reserved and serious. Somewhere around age six, her wardrobe turned black, making her the first Goth in her kindergarten class. Fortunately for her future chances for melanoma, she hates sunlight, preferring rain, clouds, and cold. Someday, she and some windswept moors are going to be very happy together. I reply to her, as honestly as I can. "I'm going to try," I say. "Really hard."

That night I have a dream. In it, it happens very quickly. We're in the kitchen—actually, it's a subconscious version of my kitchen, far bigger and cleaner than the real thing—when a woman who looks unmistakably like Gertrude Stein creeps into the room. She is holding a knife. "I'm going to kill you," she says, "and you can't stop me." I open my mouth in horror and no sound comes out. She is amused. "Look at you," she laughs. "You can't even scream." I open my mouth again, and still cannot make a sound. You have to scream, I think, you have to get help. Just do it. Scream. My knees give out from under me. I watch my children's faces go from surprise to concern to horror. As I tumble to the ground, I realize with a silent, certain helplessness, that I'm dead. But when I wake myself and the rest of the house up, I am screaming.

INTERLUDE

Cancer for Beginners

The body is a brilliant machine, designed to be strong and resilient. It heals from wounds and fends off sickness. It provides us with T cells, which patrol the body to recognize and destroy abnormalities and invaders. Most of the time, the system self-regulates without us even being aware of the work it's doing. But sometimes, the system glitches.

As Dr. Jedd Wolchok, chief of Memorial Sloan Kettering's Melanoma and Immunotherapeutics Service and the guy who eventually saved my life, explains it: "The idea is that there are several phases in immune surveillance. The first is elimination. Tumor arises. Immune system sees it. It's gotten rid of. End of story. The next phase is equilibrium, where a tumor arises, the immune system sees it, can't quite get rid of it, but the cancer doesn't do any more; it doesn't spread. Then there's the final E—escape. Escape is what we deal with, unfortunately, on a day-to-day basis. The tumor has learned skills that allow it to evade the immune system."

Cancerous cells, clever devils that they are, contain an inhibitory signal that scrambles that immune system response. That's what allows cancer to survive and the reason that cancer cells spread—the T cells that are supposed to destroy them don't know to kill them.

Once the immune system has been overridden, it's traditionally been the job of conventional—and invasive—protocols to do that work of fighting cancer instead. And once you've experienced cancer firsthand, it's generally been understood that you will live forever with the awareness that it's always lurking around the fringes of your future, waiting to pop up on the next set of scans. There's always been another shoe that could drop, another chance the signal could get scrambled again.

For generations, treatment barely progressed beyond surgery, radiation, and chemo—the holy trinity known as slash, burn, and poison. For many patients, these treatments are highly effective. But because cancer invades on a cellular level, it can be an extraordinary challenge to remove it definitively—and blasting away cancer frequently comes at the expense of the healthy parts of the body too. Surgery cuts around wide margins of the cancer's surrounding terrain. Chemo kills dividing normal cells as well as cancerous ones.

The toll both disease and its treatment extract can be profound. Writing in 1957, Australian virologist Macfarlane Burnet concluded that "there is little ground for optimism in cancer," but added that while at the time "anti-cancer drugs are also carcinogens. . . . A slightly more hopeful approach, which is, however, so dependent on the body's own resources that it has never been seriously propounded, is an immunological one."

When President Richard Nixon signed the National Cancer Act of 1971, it was the beginning of a new era in looking at how cancer behaves—and exploring new ways of treating it. Recalling it now, Dr. James Allison, professor and chair of immunology and executive director of the immunotherapy platform at MD Anderson Cancer Center, says, "The best advisers in the field said, 'We don't know much but to throw chemo and radiation and surgery at cancer.' I think what subsequently came out of that work was an amazing amount of detailed information about normal cell growth regulation and how it goes awry in cancer. It's really magnificent. All that work was essential and had to be done."

Nearly 40 years later, in 2009, the Obama Administration launched a similar initiative, vowing a broad allocation of funds toward medical research across a wide spectrum, including one billion dollars for "research into the genetic causes of cancer and potential targeted treatments." Yet even now, the default protocols for patient treatment are still often limited to the familiar trio: surgery, radiation, and chemo. And although overall cancer incidence and death rates have declined since what became known as the 1970s War on Cancer, progress has been slow and success has been erratic.

One of the other great challenges for researchers has been that cancer has an exasperatingly bountiful array of manifestations. There are more than 100 different kinds of cancer that affect humans. There are cancers of the blood and bones and organs. Cancer is many, many things, though "sneaky" and "unpredictable" tend to be among the universal traits. A big breakthrough for one form of it doesn't automatically mean a hopeful "cure" for any other types. Your neuroblastoma isn't someone else's breast cancer. The phrase "breast cancer" itself can mean different things to a person with the BRCA2 gene mutation and one without it. And because of individual circumstances and cell mutations, my melanoma isn't your melanoma.

That's why there will likely never be a cure for cancer. And I say that as someone who has, for all intents and purposes, been cured. Cancer is not a single disease, and it almost certainly can't ever be addressed with a single magical potion. It has to be approached with a variety of protocols. So when well-meaning people—or, more infuriatingly, certain cancer organizations that ought to know better—talk about finding "the cure" for "this disease," it's a good bet that they are talking a lot of nonsense. The path of medical research progress is not leading to one solution for everything. But as science moves forward with increasing sophistication and depth, there are going to be more and more patients like me: people fortunate enough to obtain a specific treatment—or combination of treatments—that seems to eradicate their cancers. Even then, though, there will probably always continue to be people for whom those same treatments simply don't work. We aren't built on assembly lines. Our bodies are unique. Our cancers are too.

CHAPTER 3

Welcome to Cancer Town

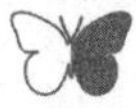

August 12, 2010

Imagine that someone woke you up in the middle of the night, put a pillowcase over your head, threw you in the trunk of a car, and then dumped you in a foreign country with the parting message, "This is where you live now." You don't speak the language. You don't know the terrain. Your new job, for whatever you may have left of your sorry life, is to figure it out. This is what the period immediately following finding out you have cancer is like.

Take, for instance, Midtown East. I'm never in this part of Manhattan. There's absolutely nothing to ever bring me here—no work commitments, no friends, and God knows no decent bars. As Jeff and I walk toward 53rd Street and 3rd Avenue this late weekday morning after dropping the kids at camp, I am painfully aware that this neighborhood of drab office buildings and coffee carts, of Duane Reade and Jamba Juice, is about to be a stranger to me no longer. I have already added Sloan Kettering to my contacts list on my phone.

In time I will learn medical terms and drug names; I'll figure out where to go for soup or a magazine too. I'll belong here. The impending familiarity of it all makes me immediately, desperately despondent. This is where I live now.

We are already approaching our destination nerve-rackingly ahead of schedule and it's almost noon—two conditions that I take as signs from the universe. "We have plenty of time for a drink," I tell Jeff. Because we don't yet know the area and don't feel like working too hard, we just duck into the café downstairs at Bloomingdale's. I order a Stoli and tonic and popovers with extra butter and give the waiter a look that says, "You want to make something of it?"

Poor Jeff. Just a few weeks ago he had a healthy dad, a healthy partner, and was enjoying plenty of healthy makeup sex. Just a few weeks ago, after a rough couple of years, things were really looking up for the guy. Now he's sitting at a table across from a woman who's trying to gauge how sober she has to stay to fathom what her new oncologist has to say, and how drunk she needs to be to hear it.

"You know," Jeff says, "cancer's not like it used to be in the old days. You might not even lose your hair. Dad didn't."

Jeff's parents live just a few miles away in the suburbs of Westchester. For 20 years, they've been the guiding parental figures of my life. My own father walked out three months before I was born, and I've only ever met him a handful of times in my life. I'm not even sure where he lives. My mother and I have a strained and distant connection. I love her, and I know she loves me. But there are mental health issues that keep us apart. We rarely speak, and even though she lives a short train ride away in New Jersey, I haven't seen her in five years. I haven't told her yet I have cancer, and I'm not sure how or if I will. You don't always get a good relationship with your parents in this life. You don't always get a relationship, period.

Jeff's folks, in contrast, took me in as one of their own from the first time I came over for dinner. Even when Jeff and I were separated, they included me in family events and treated me like a daughter. When we called them last night, we drafted them into our cancer crisis management team, because I love and trust them. And because they have experience.

Thirteen months ago, Dad was diagnosed with colon cancer during a routine checkup. He sailed through surgery and a relatively mild course of chemo, staying healthy enough along the way for vacations in Japan and Scotland. He and Jeff's mom have been everywhere, and they live to travel. The walls of their home are covered in photos and Dad's paintings from their adventures. When Dad finished chemo in March and the doctors declared him cancer free, he and Mom immediately booked a fall sightseeing journey through the national parks of the Southwest canyons.

But just last month, on his follow-up annual CT scan, the doctor saw what looked like the cancer again, spreading to his stomach. A biopsy confirmed it. He's starting a second round of chemo in September, and now the vacation will have to wait. "That's how it is with the crazy cancer," Mom had said when she called Jeff to tell him. "They think they've got it and it comes back." This time, the doctors say, the chemo is going to be more "extreme." Dad and Mom responded by planning a trip to Key West for the winter.

Dad's slowed down a lot in the past year. At 78, he's not exactly psyched about having his cancer back just a year after going through it, but he's far from grim about it. "I feel like I have a lot more things to do yet," he always says, "and I don't see why I wouldn't do them." And as a retired minister who met his wife while they were at seminary together, he has a well-mastered system for dealing with life's spiritual challenges. Jeff and I have been trying to follow his lead and remain hopeful and optimistic. About him. Now, about me too. Because I am only 44, and I have a lot of things to do as well.

I think of Dad as I pick at my popover, feeling the vodka going straight to my already adrenaline-flooded system. "When this is over,"

I say to Jeff, "I'm going to open up a bar directly across the street from Sloan Kettering, and I'm going to become a millionaire."

"I always knew you'd be my gravy train," he replies. "What are you going to call it? The Stage 4 Deli?"

"Nah," I say. "I was thinking Terminal."

After our fortifying carbohydrates and alcohol, Jeff and I make our way at last to one of the few New York City landmarks I've never visited: Memorial Sloan Kettering Cancer Center. This place is famous. It's the oldest and largest private cancer center in the world. It's the Madison Square Garden of research, the Radio City Music Hall of chemo. In the national ranking of cancer facilities, Sloan Kettering eternally races neck and neck for the top spot with Houston's MD Anderson. By virtue of my health insurance network, my dermatologist's affiliations, and the fact that I live in New York City, I have been hooked up with one of the premier treatment centers in the world. I still have malignant melanoma, but in terms of cancer care, I have hit the jackpot.

Yet even with its auspicious reputation, MSKCC is still not what I expected. Up to this point in my life, my blessedly limited experience with medical facilities has been that they're where you go to get treated like garbage when you're sick. They're where the administrators ignore you and act exasperated when you ask questions and leave you freezing on a stretcher for hours at a time. They're where harried, cranky doctors fend off crazy people in dingy emergency rooms, and Nurse Ratcheds with clipboards browbeat you about filling out your forms incorrectly. That's what I think, anyway, because that's what I've endured in the past.

This joint, in contrast, is like the nicest Marriott Marquis I've ever seen. There's soothing lighting and a waterfall wall in the lobby, and a concierge desk where the nervous newbies are directed to their destinations.

Up on the third floor, a cheerful squad of administrators greets Jeff and me as if they've been looking forward to seeing us all day and ushers us to the waiting area. There is a station of free coffee and tea, and crackers and hard candy. There are orchids and large windows and happy paintings of flowers. The last time I was anyplace like this, I was using the spa gift certificate a friend gave me for my birthday. "Yikes," I say to Jeff. "I must be in huge trouble."

The fact that everything here is easy and welcoming only serves to throw into sharp relief the palpable sense of terror in the air. There is a girl in her early 20s across from me sporting a Led Zep shirt and a peach fuzz haircut. There is an elderly couple slumped on each other on a couch. There is a middle-aged man speaking into a cell phone in clipped, authoritative Russian. None of them are crying; none are losing it. They simply emanate the urgency this space and this situation command. Outside, afternoon shadows are falling over the East Side. From my chair in the waiting room I can see straight into the building across the street, at the office workers back in the real world briskly moving around their cubicles. Do they ever look over here at us? Do they see our faces, and wonder how we got here?

A doe-eyed girl in a black sheath dress strolls into the room. "Miss Williams? Mary Williams?" she chirps brightly.

"It's Mary Elizabeth," I say. I don't want to be an abbreviated name on a form. I don't want to be a patient at all. I want someone to tell me this was just a silly mix-up and to go home now.

Instead, the manic pixie hospital admin beckons me to follow her. I wave to Jeff like I'm being led into a war crimes tribunal as she ushers me into an examination room, where she hands me a seersucker robe. Seersucker. I should have known that an East Side joint with a name like Sloan would be the preppiest hospital in the United States. I wonder if they switch to plaid flannel after Labor Day.

A few minutes later, my new oncologist, Dr. Partridge, strolls in. She has a chic bob, platinum gray hair, and a patrician manner befitting our elegant surroundings. But her eyes are lively and bright, and I sense immediately a distinctive air of mischief about her.

"Let's take a look at what we've got here," she says, pulling apart the hairs on my head and inspecting the damage. "Yup," she says simply, and my last hope that I don't belong here dissipates. "Now I need to feel your lymph nodes," she adds, and suddenly she's thrusting her hands around my neck.

This morning as I drank my coffee, I had practiced my speech. But here, in this humblingly short gown, the words don't come out so easily. "I want to tell you a few things before we move forward," I say as she prods my armpits and I squirm. "I have a family and a career and a parent with cancer, and I can't be stressing out about this too. So all I want you to tell me is what you're going to do and what I need to do. I don't need anything else. Okay?"

Her demeanor is crisp and professional. "Of course," she says, before adding, "So tell me about your kids." She thumps around my body, pushing her fingertips into my groin as I brag on about the girls, grateful for the distraction.

Then Dr. Partridge tells me, gently but emotionlessly, what I'm in for. "Your lymph nodes feel good," she says, "so my initial opinion is that this is treatable. But this is a sizable melanoma, and we're going to be very aggressive about removing it." She takes a breath, long enough for me to run the words "treatable" and "aggressive" through with the highlighter pen in my brain.

"We're going to operate," she continues, "and we have to remove around the margins as well to be safe." She grabs a pen and draws a neat circle, roughly the diameter of a good-size plum, on a piece of paper. "Based on the size and depth of your tumor, this is what we're taking off. We'll take a skin graft from another part of your body, either your neck or your thigh, then replace the skin. Do you have a preference—right or left side?" Apparently I get a say in which half of my body is harvested but not which part. Then she adds nonchalantly, "You're going to have a bald spot. The hair won't grow back. We also need to biopsy your lymph nodes, so we'll remove those from your neck. Then when we get back all the information from the surgery, we'll know how to proceed with your course of treatment."

I cling to one word. "It's treatable," I say.

"I said I believe it's treatable," she replies. I understand. No promises. No miracles. She pulls out a date book and says, "It seems like we want to get this over with soon. How's next Friday?" She says it like I'm going to say no, like I'm going to have other plans that will conflict with the removal of my malignant cancer.

This is close to what I do. "The 20th? I guess so," I reply. It's the girls' last day of camp. We usually celebrate it with a night out of Chinese food and an outdoor movie by the Hudson River. "How does this work?" I ask. "Is this an in-office procedure? Local anesthetic?"

Dr. Partridge casts a quizzical look in my direction. "Uh, no," she says. "You'll have to stay at least one night in the hospital, maybe more, depending on how the surgery goes and how you're feeling afterward."

"I see," I answer. No Chinese food or movie that night after all. "We have tickets to a Liberty game for Sunday," I continue. "Do you think I'll be able to go? Will I be back to work on Monday? Tuesday I'm taking my older daughter to see *Wicked.*"

"You're going to miss your basketball game," she tells me, patiently. "You're not going to be ready to work for a few weeks. You're going to put your feet up, and be treated like a princess for a while. You're not going to do housework; you're not going to cook; you're going to be waited on hand and foot."

Never has a promise of rest and relaxation sounded so fraught with dread. You're not going to do all the things that make your life a glorious mess, you see, because you are not a normal person anymore. You are a sick one. Your little bump on your head is not a little bump in your life. This thing is about to change all your goddamn plans. You've earned this extended staycation the worst way possible. "I guess I don't really know how this works," I say. "I've been lucky so far."

"You're right," she says as she puts her hand around my shoulder and walks me back out to the waiting room. "You were lucky." Were.

That night Jeff and I sit the kids on the couch and tell them the plan we hastily hatched on the subway ride home. "Next week, I'm going to the hospital for a night or two so they can take my cancer out," I say. "You're still going to camp, and then you'll go out to Grandma and Grandpa's for the night. When you come back, I'll need some time to recover, and I'll have a bald spot on my head, but I'll still be Mom."

My firstborn, ever practical, has a few questions. The primary one is "Who's going to do my laundry?"

"I'm going to take care of everything," Jeff says, and Lucy looks utterly appalled.

"You'll be out of the hospital in time for us to go to *Wicked,* right?" she presses further.

"The doctor says I won't be well enough yet to go out. Daddy's going to take you," I explain. "And Grandma will stay here to help me take care of Bea."

That's when both of my children start crying at the horrible unfairness of it all. "You and I were going to go!" Lucy sobs.

"Daddy and I were going to order a pizza!" Bea pouts.

The idea that Mom has cancer, a disease my children only vaguely understand as the thing Grandpa had to get an operation and treatment for, is incredibly abstract. But Mommy not doing laundry, not taking them to shows? Now, that's serious.

"No," Lucy says through angry tears. "I don't want Daddy to do my laundry, and I don't want Daddy to take me to *Wicked.*"

"I'm sad too," I say. "Maybe when I'm all better, you and I can go too?"

"Okay," she says reluctantly. I suspect the most expensive part of my cancer treatment will end up being all the bribes I'll have to give my kids.

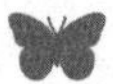

After the children are sufficiently reassured and sent to bed, I climb into my own and turn on my laptop. Less than an hour later I have poured out the story of the past two days—the shock of the news, the hope for better times to come. I read over what I have written, and impulsively send an email to my Salon editor, Thomas. "You can publish this if you want," I say. "I just needed to write it."

I then send an email to my college roommates Debbie and Jill, and Jill's wife Michele. It reads: "So I have a malignant melanoma on my scalp and am having surgery next week. Once we biopsy my lymph nodes, I'm probably starting chemo. I still fully plan on continuing to play with you guys as much as humanly possible. But you three are right up near the top of my list of most important people in my life and I wanted to let you know what's going on. And to tell you this means you have to buy me drinks. I love you."

After work the next day, I ride the subway downtown for a last day of camp dinner, one week ahead of schedule. As Jeff and the girls and I pick over the last of the Chinese food, I look out the window of Sammy's, savoring the way the waning sunlight hits the brick buildings and the beautiful people strolling by. I love New York City best in the late summer, when it's hot and sticky and all the publicists and shrinks have left town. But now I'd really love to see it in the fall. It's been only two days, but I'm already grieving for the person I was on August 10. Her unquestioning ability to plan things far in advance, her unshakeable certainty of her own future existence, her ability to walk down Broadway on a bright summer day with no hat and no fear. She was obliterated in the span of a phone call. I wish I'd had a chance to say goodbye.

By the time the kids are asleep, I'm exhausted, but I can't resist checking on Salon. There on the front page is my face, looking wry and skeptical, above the words "My cancer diagnosis." I have a headache just considering the implications of what I have just irreversibly done. But since the news is out anyway, I do the next logical thing. I click on the share button at the bottom of the page, and send it out via Twitter and Facebook. In one small motion of my finger, I inform a legion of friends, a pack of colleagues, a fair number of total strangers, and perhaps even, somewhere, my own parents, that I have malignant cancer. That, folks, is how you rip off a Band-Aid.

CHAPTER 4

Off the Top of My Head

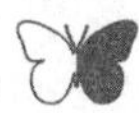

August 15, 2010

My last Sunday with an intact head is a glorious one for the family to go to Governors Island. It's one of my favorite spots in the city, an oasis of trees and beautiful views and quirky public art plunked right off the edge of Manhattan. I eat nachos for lunch, washed down with beer and zero regret. Afterward, we all rent bicycles, and as we pedal around the circumference of the island, it doesn't take long for Bea's patience with pedestrians to run out. As we creak toward a particularly thick throng, she bellows, "Outta the way! My mom has cancer!"

I turn my head back at her. The wind is blowing through her long hair, and she is laughing uproariously. "Outta the way!" she repeats. Then Lucy joins in. "Our mom has cancer, everybody!" In case you ever need to disperse a crowd, I can report that this gambit works like a charm.

Later, on the subway ride home, Bea curls up next to me and falls asleep on my shoulder. Her tender, trusting nature is so pure it floors me on a daily basis. As the fussed-over baby of our family, she assumes the world will adore her, and takes applause as her due. What's impressive about her is how much love she gives right back. She is lavish in her affections, dispensing hugs generously and scattering love notes to the rest of us around the apartment. My sunny sweetie. How little pain and worry you've had in your short life. How little I hope to trouble you now.

How little I have ever wanted to trouble anybody, really. My headstone will likely read: "I'm fine. Whatever." But now I am in a pickle, the serious kind, and as the days approaching my surgery dwindle down, a new dynamic between my friends and me has emerged. A seismic shift occurred the moment I shared my diagnosis, and when the ground stopped moving, my relationships had been rearranged. Some people—people I never doubted would be there through thick and thin—have been conspicuously avoiding me, and worse, avoiding the kids. Others have unhelpfully regaled me with their own horror stories and anxieties. Many others have been supremely great, though, with greatness specific to their generous souls. Jill and Michele have offered to come up from Miami. Carolyn has sent jars of homemade jams and pickles. Martin has magnanimously told me that if I need any extra help during recovery, he's got "two dead parents and all their pills." Ben has cheerfully volunteered his medical marijuana card and added, "Wig sex is hot. Like you don't already know." Stephanie—a vegetarian—has dropped by with three meat loaves. Anne, a cancer veteran herself, has advised, "Don't Google worst-case scenarios. Keep positive people close. Remember that most of us live."

My favorite response is from my colleague King, because King knows. In January, he fell suddenly and seriously ill with a rare, potentially life-altering disorder known as Guillain-Barré. He spent several weeks in the hospital and for a while didn't know if he would ever regain the use of his limbs. It was a scary time, one he recovered from with odds-defying speed. Naturally, he has written competitively to me, "This was my year, bitch." In the next line, he's added, "I've discovered the answer to 'Why?' is 'Because,' and the answer to 'Why me?' is 'Why not you?' So let people do astonishingly generous things for you. Know why? Because why not you?"

Then there's Debbie.

Debbie is the Tina Fey character of my life. Pretty, dark-haired, and bespectacled, she is married to her college sweetheart, teaches elementary school, has two sons named Tim and Adam, and has never strayed far from the Philadelphia suburb where she grew up. She also has the filthiest mouth and the most punk rock sensibility of any human being I have ever encountered. So when a large box with a Pennsylvania postmark arrives in the mail, I know its provenance immediately. In the box are two dozen homemade chocolate chip cookies with a note that says, "Rich in antioxidants!" There is also a T-shirt in my favorite shade of green. Debbie designed it herself. It reads: FUCK CANCER.

On the morning before my surgery, I put on my shorts and my sports bra and sneakers and run around the park, as I do most mornings. This time, however, is the last time for a long time, so I run as if an ax murderer is chasing me. I run five miles at a crushing pace, the Beastie Boys blaring in my ears, drowning out the sound of my increasingly hard breathing. I'm shoring up endorphins, determined to make this the sweetest, sweatiest run of the summer.

That evening is trivia night at the local bar, and it's a beautiful night for a send-off among friends. Our team, the self-explanatorily named Mothers Who Drink, does respectably in local history and sci-fi films. And when the category turns to Harry Potter, the table full of moms is raging.

When we wind up tied with another team, it prompts a sudden-death match—a chugging competition. "Who's representing the Mothers?" the MC hoots to our table. Everyone points at me. This will be the last thing I consume before my surgery. Might as well make it worthwhile.

My male adversary is younger and bigger, but tonight, I've got the eye of the tiger. On the count of three, I pour the pint down my throat in one big gulp, bringing glory and a commemorative T-shirt back for the team. You gotta fight. For your right. To paaaaaaarrrtay.

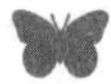

August 20, 2010

It's well before dawn, and I am luxuriating in a long shower, scrubbing my hair, and running my fingers along my still intact scalp. Occasionally I glide over the bump. Hello, cancer, I think. Your time here is up.

My bag is packed with my favorite pajamas, a copy of Lev Grossman's *The Magicians,* the newest issue of *InStyle,* and a handmade card that says "I LOVE YOU MOM" in a six-year-old's scrawl. I slip into the black jersey dress I wore to visit my friend Larry and his wife in Barcelona last September. When I told him last week I had cancer, he'd replied, "You and me, dancing all night in Spain, ten years from today." Every time I look at that dress I think of the Sagrada Família, and the three-hour lunch by the beach, and the gay tapas bar in the Gothic Quarter. Now it's my going to cancer surgery dress.

Jeff opens his eyes reluctantly and waves at me as I pick up the bag. We're working very hard to keep things normal here. He's taking the girls to their final day of camp this morning, and picking them up this afternoon. We both want them to have this day, and for my cancer to not get in the way of it. "See you around, babe," I say. "Your money's on the dresser." I peek in on the girls, snug in their bunks.

Lucy groggily sits up in her bed. "Mommy," she says, smiling proudly. I strongly suspect she willed herself to wake up at this unholy hour just to send me off. "You have a great last day of camp," I tell her, and I kiss her sleepy, rumpled head.

Minutes later, my cab is careering down the FDR Drive as the day is breaking over Manhattan. I spend much of the ride mussing my still damp tresses and smoothing them out again. After today, that experience will never be the same. There will be an empty patch on the top of my head where no hair will ever grow again. Outside, the early crowd is bustling to work, grabbing their coffees and bagels from the corner carts. It's the rhythm of life, pulsing on, just outside this building, teeming with folks in various stages of cancer, that I'm racing toward. I find solace in that.

At the hospital, I while away the morning staring out the window, trying to memorize every detail I see outside, because illogically, I think that if this were to be my last day on Earth, I would want to remember it. I read the same page of *The Magicians* over and over without a word of it sinking in. I eavesdrop on the patient next to me, a chubby middle-aged man in for prostate surgery. "Things are changing all the time," his doctor says brightly to the lady I assume is his wife. "Cancer used to be a lot scarier. We're now looking at it as a long-term condition that can be managed." I'm beginning to understand that cancer is no longer exclusively something you triumph over, Robin Roberts style, or slowly die of, Warren Zevon style. It could instead be something you learn to live with.

In the world I too lived in just a few weeks ago, people talk about cancer as if being entirely disease free is the only measure of a healthy, satisfying life. But in here, in Cancer Town, success is often measured not in terms of disease going entirely away, but by simple survival. How can you say who's officially "cured" without knowing 100 percent what's happening in every cell in a person's body anyway? Even scans can't do that. What if treatment succeeds only as far as shrinking the tumors? What if it only arrests their growth? There's no snappy T-shirt slogan to be had, no "Race for the Cessation of Progression." To have the cancer go away entirely is great. It's exactly what I hope for today. But in the all-or-nothing magical thinking around cancer, no one admits that the word "cure" doesn't encompass the breathtaking, beautiful possibility of living, living well and living long, with cancer in your body. You can survive and never be "cured." Turns out it happens all the time. That would be plenty good enough for me.

Around midday, Dr. Edwards, the surgical assistant, lopes in to introduce himself. Dr. Edwards is a big, bearded, rumpled man who looks like a cross between a professor and a bass guitarist. "I have to draw on you now," he says gently, as he stipples his pen along my left thigh and the left side of my neck.

His voice is soothing, even if I don't understand most of what he's saying. Stuff about incisions and sutures. "When you get into the OR, your nurse will be Alan. You're going to love Alan," he says.

"I can't wait to meet him," I reply.

"Then I think it's just about showtime," he says, in the same comforting tone he's used throughout. He pats me on the back. "Let's go kick some ass."

A half hour later the orderly comes for me. "You ready?" he asks. Back on January 1, I made a New Year's resolution. Thanks to my pal Larry and his infectious mania for turning everything into a six-word story, I had distilled my goal for the year 2010 into a half dozen–worded plan: Go somewhere I've never been before. Okay. So let's go.

There's no dramatic ride on a stretcher, like in the movies. There's just me in a seersucker gown and a shower cap and silly booties, dragging an IV pole as the orderly walks me down an endless corridor, past several sets of doors and several sets of surgeries. The air grows exponentially colder the farther we go. I wonder if that's why I'm trembling uncontrollably.

Then I'm in the room. There's the table. My table. There are Dr. Partridge and Dr. Edwards and a handful of nurses. They're all wearing masks. I feel at once exposed and underdressed, like Tom Cruise at that orgy in *Eyes Wide Shut*. A masked man steps forward to guide me. "I'm Alan," he says.

"I've heard so much about you," I reply, making small talk at our party with ridiculous costumes and much too assertive air-conditioning.

My eyes sweep over a tray of gleaming instruments as I hop gracelessly onto the table and onto my back. Alan fiddles with my IV port. "We're going to give you a cocktail of sedatives before the anesthesia," Dr. Edwards explains. "It's standard." Then he adds, "I've already had a few cocktails myself."

Dr. Partridge leans in over my face and deadpans, "It steadies his hands." My surgical team at one of the world's most prestigious cancer hospitals. What a bunch of cutups, I think. I don't even feel my eyes close.

I awaken in the operating room. It feels abrupt, like an alarm going off, and I resent the interruption of my dreams. I can feel the gurney rolling me down a corridor. I am drowsy and distinctly aware that I am still doped to the gills. I am conscious of someone taking me somewhere new and parking me in a dimly lit corner of a room. Just let me go back to sleep. Let me sleep. How can a lady get any rest around here with all this chatting, and right at the foot of my bed?

"How are you feeling?" asks my nurse, who looks so much like Edie Falco's Nurse Jackie that my druggy brain is convinced she is Nurse Jackie. I don't know yet. Mostly I am gripped with an increasingly terrifying awareness, like a character in one of the Saw movies, of just how much freaky apparatus I'm tethered to. My calves, for instance, are enrobed in what look like balloons. *Puff puff puff chhhhhhhhh*. They inflate with air. *Hisssss.* They flatten. It's to keep the blood flowing through my legs, presumably so I don't get an embolism and die. There's also a clip attached to my forefinger that measures my heart rate. There's an IV drip in my arm. The bed undulates every few minutes to keep my circulation going and prevent bedsores. There's blood seeping out from underneath a bandage on my left thigh. My head, meanwhile, feels so heavy. That's when I understand that it is swaddled in bandages. They're wrapped up all around me like a thick cocoon. Oh God, they really did it. They operated on me. I think it hurts.

"How do you feel?" Nurse Jackie asks again. I blink at her questioningly. How do I feel? Like I just had the top of my head sliced off, I guess.

"Hungry," I reply.

She gives me a sly nod. "I've got a menu right here at my station," she says. She hands me a list of words called a "menu" and a "pen," but I am still far too gone to remember what one does with such things. I crudely check off the box next to the words "turkey burger" and slur, "I'd like to see the wine list."

Dr. Partridge is standing at my side. How long has she been there? "The surgery went fine," she says. "I left a message for Jeff. I think it was Jeff, I couldn't tell from the outgoing voice mail. He should be on his way soon. Or somebody else with the number you gave me." Then she's not there. I am seriously high right now.

With spectacular effort, of which I am heroically proud, I manage to pull my television set close and flick it on. My favorite of the Harry Potter movies, *Goblet of Fire,* is on. A few minutes later, Jeff arrives. I'm in the first bed in the ward and I'm the one with a turban of bandages, so he can't miss me. "The girls had a great last day of camp," he says. "They send their love." I wish I could call them, but I'm scarily incoherent.

"Hey, remember how you wanted to get back together?" I mumble. "Sucker, you were almost free. Bet you didn't think I'd pull this. Now you have to stick with me or everyone will think you're an asshole like Newt Gingrich."

"Well played," he says.

"Sit down," I say. "It's Harry Potter. You can be my Friday night date." He eases into the chair next to me and holds my hand until it's time to move me to my room, and he has to leave. I am still very dopey as he stands in our impossibly brightly lit hallway and waves goodbye to me as I roll away. But I am with it enough to recognize the look on his face. It's profound sadness.

I don't really sleep that night. I instead spend the evening pushing my IV tower to the bathroom every time I have to pee and having nice strangers come in and change my bloody bedclothes and sheets and give me painkillers. But the hours slip by, and eventually, while lavender dawn creeps over the 59th Street Bridge, I feel myself fade off into dreamless slumber.

I am awakened much too early in the morning by two strangers named Dr. Balthazar and Dr. Stewart. One of them, they explain as they take my vitals, is the resident and one of them is the fellow, and I don't know what either of those terms means anyway.

"We've made your appointment to come back and meet with Dr. Partridge. In the meantime, we're going to give you a prescription for Percocet," Dr. Stewart informs me. "We're having it filled now so you can take it with you. You should pick up some stool softeners on the way home." He glances up from my chart to look me over. "Percocet can be very constipating." There is no dignity. There is just no dignity.

A few groggy hours later, I'm being pronounced well enough for discharge, and Jeff and I are in the backseat of my friend Shannon's car, hauling ass back home. Home. Jeff opens up the black front door to the apartment we spent three years searching for. The place where our children sleep. I feel like I've been gone away a lifetime. It's eerily empty without the kids, who are still safely ensconced with Jeff's parents in White Plains. On the dining table is a lush floral arrangement from my co-workers at Salon. The card reads, "Good luck telling cancer to go fuck itself. From your family."

Though I have what I believe is plenty of my own steam, Jeff protectively ushers me directly into the bedroom, which he has specially prepared for my convalescence. The bed is turned down on my side, and Bea's pink bolster is propped up on it. A folding table is perched nearby for all my beverage, book, and pharmaceutical needs. "This looks so good," I tell him as I crawl in. "Thank you." Then I fall asleep so quickly and so deeply I don't remember anything else for a long time.

I am napping my way through the afternoon when Jeff's mom returns the kids, but I groggily rouse when I hear the dainty rumble of their feet excitedly pounding their way through the bedroom door. I slowly hoist myself up. My head is still wrapped in bandages and topped with a jaunty mesh cap, knotted at the top. I look like a cross between Little Edie and a Keebler elf.

"You need to be very gentle with Mommy," says Jeff, and they slow down right in mid-pounce, their faces going from giddy to solemn as they take in the sight of their bandaged, messy mom. Fortunately, all my procedures are on the left part of my body. "Just don't get on my bad side," I reply, beckoning them toward me for a modified hug. Then I command, "Come with me," and drag myself out of bed and march into their bedroom.

I dig out the girls' overstuffed bin of assorted magic markers in various states of inky viability and their dress-up shopping bag of ribbons and pieces of lace, and dump the lot on the dining table next to my pile of fresh mesh caps.

"The nurses said I need you to decorate them," I say.

"That's so fun," Bea says, her eyes lighting up at the prospect of a project. "This is the funnest thing that happened since you got cancer. You've got to be okay if we can do this." Then she adds, more gravely, "I guess this is a big deal, right?" Yeah, I'm still processing that one myself.

We spread our notions out and set to bedazzling my headgear. We thread delicate ribbons through the mesh weave. We draw flowers and butterflies. Bea festoons a cap with bright green lace, and Lucy monograms my name in script. We thread and knot and tie cute bows. Combined with the hot pink Lilly Pulitzer beach cover-up I'm rocking, the eccentric invalid motif is now complete. I put on one of my caps.

"What do you think?" I ask.

"You don't look sick, Mommy," Bea says approvingly. "You just look crazy."

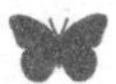

That night, nauseatingly drugged out on Percocet and exhausted, I turn in early while Jeff stays up watching *Billy Madison* for the umpteenth time. It's not even 11 p.m. when I rouse from a deep sleep and stumble to the bathroom for a pee run. I drowsily wash my hands, and then absently sweep my hair off my shoulders. As I do so, I touch my neck. My knees are buckling underneath me.

It isn't even a thought yet. I've just felt the place they biopsied my lymph nodes, and it's swollen either from the procedure or something far more serious. Is that a tumor? Is that what one feels like? It doesn't matter right now anyway, because the room is going black around me. I'm hyperventilating now, lurching toward a perch on the edge of the toilet while I feebly call out for help. "Jeff?" I moan. "Something's wrong."

Through the fog, I feel his cool hand guide me toward the bed, where I crash like I've been dropped from a great height. I hear his voice, muffled, speaking from far away. "Just breathe with me, okay?" he says. "One, two, three, inhale. Four, five, six, exhale. Good girl."

So this is an anxiety attack. This is what it's like when the darkest part of your brain takes your body hostage.

"You're doing fine," Jeff coos soothingly as I frantically continue to attempt to remember how to breathe. I hear his footsteps tread out of the room and soon after approach again. I feel a washcloth on my brow. If the cancer doesn't kill me, the hysteria may do it first.

CHAPTER 5

Don't Call Me a Survivor

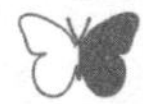

September 2010

I'm sure that every minute you're waiting for the lab results from your cancer surgery always feels interminable, but no joke, the wait at Sloan Kettering today is ridiculous.

For my first postsurgery doctor's appointment, I am today wearing the bright green FUCK CANCER shirt that Debbie gave me with a flowing peasant skirt, an item chosen because it seemed the least likely thing in my wardrobe to rub up against the bandaged, playing card–size patch on my thigh where my skin used to be. My head is still swaddled in bandages and my little mesh elf cap. I feel impossibly fragile, like I'm balancing a newborn on my head. As I shift uncomfortably in my chair, I am keenly aware of the steady throbs of pain coming from several regions of my body that my first big outing since surgery has set off. Not so mighty now, are you, Percocet?

I leaf unconvincingly through a copy of *People,* trying not to notice the wig brochures fanned out on the coffee table, as Jeff makes light, jokey chitchat. I am increasingly panicky and headachy and sore and sweating like a beast. Now I know why they call it "clinical strength" deodorant. It's because it's what you need when you're waiting for your clinic results.

Finally, someone calls my name. "Mary Williams?"

"Mary Elizabeth," I say dully. I get up and wave meekly to Jeff as I trudge off to change into seersucker.

This morning, as I left for Sloan Kettering, Bea had thrown her arms around me and said, "Don't worry, Mom, the worst is over." Now I try to read Dr. Partridge's expression when she walks in the door, to determine if Bea was correct. But Dr. Partridge has the poker face down pat. So I state again what I told her on our first meeting. "Please don't tell me what stage I am. Just tell me how we're going to treat it from here."

"Then I suppose you don't want to know that the cancer wasn't in your lymph nodes?" she asks, with obvious pleasure.

"I guess you can tell me that," I tell her.

"Your margins were clean, too. It doesn't look like there's any spreading," she continues. "We don't recommend chemo for you, based on how the surgery went and because we find chemo isn't very successful as an initial course for melanoma anyway. I'd be very skeptical of anyone who tells you otherwise."

There is currently only one FDA-approved single-agent chemo drug for melanoma, dacarbazine. It has at best a 20 percent response rate in patients with late-stage melanoma—and as low as a 5 percent one. Even in people it works on, the duration of its effectiveness is often short-lived, usually only six months or fewer. Yet in 2010, it still remains the standard protocol for most patients with advanced melanoma. It's also been associated with the development of secondary malignancies. Temodar, an oral chemo drug used for brain tumors, has also been used for metastatic melanoma patients, and with similarly discouraging overall results. As one of my nurses will later recall,

"When I came to melanoma, patients were getting Temodar like Tic Tacs—and it really wasn't doing much prolonging their lives."

"You do have the option of interferon," she says, "if you feel that you want additional treatment, but we don't suggest it and don't offer it. The data don't support its effectiveness, and the side effects are awful. You'd feel like you had the flu for about a year, and it might not do any good at all. If you want to pursue it, we'd help you transfer to another care facility."

Interferons are proteins that can be used therapeutically to trigger immune system responses. The treatment has had some, but very limited, effectiveness in treating melanoma. And though Dr. Partridge doesn't mention it, interferon can also often induce or worsen depression, sometimes severely, in many patients.

"Okay," I say. "I'll think about it and let you know."

"Great," she says. "In the meantime, I'm going to make an appointment for you with our immunology team to discuss any possible adjuvant therapy they might recommend for you, and you'll come back in October for an MRI and CT scan. For now, you're cancer free. You know," she adds, "this is a terrific time in melanoma research."

I'm apparently cancer free and picked the right time to get melanoma, but my cancer was definitely not messing around. My medical report confirms that I had what has been classified as a T4b scalp melanoma with ulceration and a Clark level of 5—which means it was bigger than four millimeters in thickness, that the epidermis covering the melanoma was not intact, and that the melanoma had invaded into the subcutaneous tissue. The long-term prognosis for melanoma patients with ulceration is typically worse than those without. My cancer was, as Bea would say, a big deal. On the upside, I had a negative sentinel lymph node, and the hope is they got that big old ulcerated cancer out, and I can move on.

"So at what point," I ask her, "do you think I get to call myself a cancer survivor?"

She gives me an indulgent look and answers truthfully. "When you die of something else. Now," she adds as she gingerly begins to cut away at the bandages, "let's take a look at how we're doing." The sound of metal slicing through fabric, through the protective layer of stitching sewn to my skin, is close in my ear. The nurse dabs at my head, and then I feel a shocking trickle of cool fluid flow down to my ears. My first thought is that she's popped something disgusting, but it's just a saline solution to clean my wound. A discarded patch is tossed onto a silver tray. It is deep crimson, ringed with spiky black threads that look like the hairs on a spider's legs.

"Okaaaaay," Dr. Partridge singsongs, like you do to a child when you're about to tell her the cat died, "I can see by the pus that we've got an infection here." If I can't clear up this infection, the implication is clear—another graft surgery. Another mining of my flesh. "I'm going to give you a prescription for an oral antibiotic and some Silvadene cream," she continues. "You're going to need to clean it twice a day. If you can use saline solution, that'd be best." Before surgery, I hadn't really considered the management of my gross healing process or what that would entail. Now I understand that it's just another part of my new job in my new town. I watch Dr. Partridge intently cleaning and realize that Jeff's just been recruited too.

My nurse Nina has been standing by patiently during this whole exchange, looking at me like I'm a safe she'd like to crack open. As soon as Dr. Partridge gives her the signal, she swoops in. "We need to clean up along the edges," she says. She purses her lips as she surveys the area, and only once she's got the lay of the land does she begin to excavate it with an intimidating, tweezerlike tool. "Is that a suture?" she asks, plucking a waxy length of thick black thread out of my head and holding it up for me to inspect. Christ, I hope that's a suture. Pick, pick, pick. Dig, dig, dig. I sit stock-still as she removes packed-on ointment and God knows what else, and then proudly displays the results to me. "See that?" she says, showing off a tiny tray full of accumulated dried skin and blood. "You need to get that." Between the sight of my surgical detritus and the opioids I'm on, I feel like barfing.

Then a flash of inspiration hits Nina. She flies out of the room, and when she returns, she is carrying a fistful of plastic wands the length of chopsticks, each topped with what resembles a mascara brush. "Let's give this a try," she says, and she tenderly flicks more flakes off my head. She seems pleased with her ingenuity—and I'm absurdly grateful for a less crusty head. "You don't want to know what we really use these for," she says as she pops the bunch in a plastic bag marked BIOHAZARD and hands it to me. Let's see . . . they're long and slender . . . oh.

My margins are clean. My lymph nodes are clear. My doctor says I am cancer free. I don't need any further treatment. And just to recap, I have spent the morning having my wide-open head worked over with a cervical sampler brush.

"And how are your bowels?" Dr. Partridge asks as Nina reswaddles my melon in cream and gauze. "Is the Percocet making you constipated?"

"Outrageously," I answer truthfully. This woman has sawed open my head. I can't imagine there's any mystery left. "The stool softeners aren't cutting it."

"Move on to something stronger, then," she says, ordering me to up my laxative game, and with that imperative, I am free to leave. There is still work to be done. More doctor visits and consults and the fear of what they might reveal. My head hurts and my wounds are nowhere near healed. But there's today. There's me getting to tell my kids I don't have cancer anymore. Today is tremendous.

Later in the afternoon, when Jeff is getting ready to go get the groceries for dinner, he asks, "Do you need me to pick up anything for you while I'm out?" I decide that this is a good moment for the private concerns the doctor raised to now be shared.

"As a matter of fact, yes. I need something to help me, you know . . ." I say as my voice trails off meaningfully, "go."

"Gotcha," he replies with an exaggerated wink, and dashes off like he's a constipation-fighting superhero. When he returns a half hour later, he is beaming—and proudly carrying a full case of Fleet enemas.

"Oh sweet Lord in heaven," I say. "What have you done? How are we ever going to show our faces in the Rite Aid again?" I gaze in horror at the economy-size collection of anal paraphernalia. "They're going to think you run a fetish club now."

"You said you needed something," he shrugs. "They didn't have any individual boxes."

"I meant something in a pink box with the words 'gentle' and 'overnight' on the label, not a lifetime supply of colon hoses," I reply. He looks crestfallen. I'd given him an important mission and now I'm being ungrateful. "I'm sorry," I say. "Thank you for the case of enemas."

"You're quite welcome, my special lady," he replies. Ever the gentleman.

That evening, I flip the toilet lid down and take a seat as Jeff washes his hands and snaps on a pair of surgical gloves for his first go at cleaning the wound site. "Now, how should I do this?" he asks.

"Dr. Partridge said we should try to get something with saline," I reply. "I should have asked when you went to the drug store." Then the lightbulb goes off above what's left of my head. "Something in a squirt bottle," I continue. "That'd be convenient." I get up, go to the closet, and pull out a Fleet bottle. "Here you go, pal," I say as I hand it to him. "I think you may just be a genius."

I sit back down and he slowly pulls away the gauze padding. It's all very Bride of Frankenstein. I feel there ought to be lightning and lots of *bzzt bzzt* sounds and Jeff shouting, "She's alive! ALIVE!"

Instead, once all the bandages are off, he just quietly says, "That is intense." And he doesn't say anything else.

I get up, wordless as well. I take the hand mirror from the basket by the sink and stand in front of the medicine cabinet mirror—and do nothing. What kind of wuss are you? I think. Scared of your own body. Just look at it. Look at it. Then I bend my chin into my chest and hold up the smaller mirror behind my head so I can view, for the first time, the empty place where my hair used to be. My disaster area.

Then I gag, my breakfast bolting toward my throat. Okay, that was some serious Ray Liotta in *Hannibal* fare. Some Lucy Liu in *Kill Bill* action. What the hell happened to the top of my head? It's gone. I steady the mirror in my hand, and look again.

I know, intellectually, that this isn't my brain I'm looking at, but I'd been expecting a lot more in the way of skin up there. Below the waist, it sure looks and feels like they took plenty off my thigh. Yet up on top there's a delicate, near invisible webbing growing over blood and muscle and goo surrounding my skull and, oh my God, I might faint. I can see straight down into everything normally protected by scalp and hair. Jeff was right. That's intense.

Ever since the surgery, I'd been trying to avoid grieving for the patch of my head that's never coming back. I had thought I'd easily slip into the role of positive, cheery cancer "survivor." Instead, here it all comes now, all the darkness, flooding in all at once. It's different from the fear of cancer, or the pain of healing, although those things are still very much kicking up a storm in my psyche too. This is something else—it's straight-up loss. Of course I'm grateful the melanoma is gone, but part of my body is part of my past now, and it's odd how viscerally it affects me. I sit down on the edge of the tub, gulping air and sobbing.

I look up at Jeff. He looks both defeated and terribly tender. This is a new kind of intimacy between us—and a new kind of distance too. I'm the one who got cancer. He's the one who has to pick up the pieces. He's the one who took the kids back-to-school shopping, the one making dinner and doing the dishes, every day, and running out for enemas. I got abducted to Cancer Town, but he has chosen to come with me into it. "You ready?" he says, and continues his new job as the person in charge of my bloody, pus-filled surgical wounds. I nod, and he spackles thick white cream on my wide-open head, more delicate than an infant's fontanel, with a tongue depressor.

"I'm sorry," I say. "This sucks for you. This isn't what you signed up for when we got together."

"True," he replies. "I just wanted your roast chicken again. Still, you're not getting rid of me that easily this time." He puts his hand on my shoulder. "When you got diagnosed," he says, "I thought, this is bad. But your doctor says you're cancer free, and you don't have to have any chemo. It's gone even better than we could have hoped. What's a little spackling? Now tell me how this feels." I sense cool cream sliding over the place my scalp used to be, and the touch of someone very sweet. "It feels good," I say. It does.

The next morning is a Saturday, but sleeping in never seems to happen when you've got two young kids. Today is no different. The sun's barely up when the girls come bounding in to the bedroom from whatever cannon they've been shot out of, jumping on the bed in a pile of giggles, deftly attacking only my right side. My eyes blink open reluctantly. The girls are demanding attention, chanting, "Wake up! You're cancer free! You're cancer free!" as they smother me in kisses. Now this I can get up for.

I've still barely been outside yet, but today, we're off to visit Jeff's parents in the burbs for the first time since my surgery—and only the second time since Dad got rediagnosed. Dad looks tired but happy when I come in to the house and hug him, hug him there in the living room lined with his paintings of flowers and mountains and trees. "How are you feeling?" he asks. "Now, are you going to be getting chemo like me?"

"No chemo," I say. "Nothing else for now. I still have to meet with the immunotherapy doctor, but I don't even know what that would involve."

"Oh, that's so fortunate," he says, and I can tell he's anxious about starting treatment again. He looks more worried this time than last. I know he's trying not to let it get to him, determined not to let it interfere with his artwork and his busy schedule of museum trips and volunteer work and seeing friends. Nevertheless, it's an aggressive regimen.

Later, when I rise from the afternoon nap that the kids' early morning assault and the pain meds have made necessary, I find Dad out on the back porch with the girls. The three of them are patiently painting watercolors of a vase of gerbera daisies that perches on the table in front of them. It's a nice afternoon for painting.

When I groggily ask how he's been doing, he says, "The doctor says my numbers are good. You know, chemo's not so bad. It's mostly just boring. I'll bring a book. Or write in my journal." I imagine he has a lot of pages yet to fill.

The rest of my recuperative days pass in a blurry haze. Friends continue to generously bring over meals, dishes that my daughters fussily push around their plates. "Why did our mom have to be the one to get cancer?" Bea pouts in contempt at a neighbor's chicken potpie. I, on the other hand, am stunned by all this kindness, humbled, and a little uncomfortable with it. It's strange to let people be so nice. It's strange to be so taken care of. I used to think I was strong because I could fend for myself. I didn't know how much of a challenge it would be to surrender control like this. Come to think of it, I have always made a terrible submissive. The lesson of cancer appears to be getting me in touch with my inner power bottom.

Jeff and I have fallen into an elaborate maintenance routine. There's a folding table now in the bathroom, full of all our supplies—the squirt enema bottle and the gauze and the cream and surgical gloves and the meds. I hate it. It all makes me feel sick and old, like my grandmother at the end, propped up on pillows, surrounded by pill bottles. Twice a day, either Jeff or my nurse friend Jolie, who stops by on her way to her grueling shifts at the hospital like it's no inconvenience, will bust out the Fleet and clean my scalp, anoint it with a layer of Silvadene cream, and then cover it with a protective pillow of gauze and a head scarf. Then I get a modified version of the same procedure on my thigh. Despite all the precautions, in the mornings, I sometimes wake up smeared in blood. But while I'm still in a lot of pain, it's getting better every day, and the bottle of 30 Percocet I'd been granted is dwindling. "Are you going to save some pills for a rainy day?" my stoner friend Tad asks one afternoon as we sit in the park together, watching squirrels. I just had major surgery involving three different parts of my body, Tad, I think. I can't imagine there will come a time when I could possibly enjoy narcotics as much as I do right now.

My hair, meanwhile, is not exactly filthy, but it's definitely been roughing it. Hygiene has to be approached with the utmost of caution. Every two or three days, Jeff helps me shampoo, taking extra care around the surgical scar. I sit in the bathtub as he leans over me, helping me to suds up while avoiding the wound, and pouring fresh water from a plastic cup to rinse. Think Redford and Streep in *Out of Africa,* but gross and full of blood, and instead of Africa, it's a cramped Manhattan bathroom. Blow-drying is not even a remote possibility.

I still don't like to see my head or touch it or acknowledge it exists. I can, however, smell it clearly—and it doesn't smell like a nasty infection at all. It smells clean and earthy, like a sweet sort of sweat, like sex after a shower. "We still have some pus today," Jolie soothingly relays to me one early morning, en route to work, adding with a loving sigh, "but your granulation is beautiful. Now what's this dark business here at the edges? I can't tell if it's scabbing or necrosis. Don't worry about it." I have a beautifully granulating, sexy smelling, large, infected head wound with flesh that may or may not be dying. It's all going so well.

October 2010

I am back at Sloan Kettering this morning for post-recovery MRI and CT scans, and a brief consultation with Dr. Esposito, one of the hospital immunologists. As a newbie to cancer, I am still unfamiliar with its protocols and treatments, so I don't get that this is not an especially typical experience for someone who's recently dealt with melanoma. I don't get that having a meeting with one's immunology team is unique—because having an immunology team at all is unique—or that I am dealing with a crazy-smart group of individuals who've spent the past several years developing innovative treatments, many of which are not even available to the general market.

I don't know yet that the current chair of immunologic studies at MSKCC is James Allison, or that Allison is basically the rock star of immunotherapy—so much of a rock star, in fact, that he sings and plays harmonica in a group called the Checkpoints. I don't know that his team's work in uncovering the intricacies of a protein called cytotoxic T-lymphocyte antigen-4—or more familiarly, CTLA-4—is currently paving the way for the biggest breakthrough in melanoma treatment in decades. I just know I'm here to meet with Dr. Esposito, because Dr. Partridge said so, and that I am going to get a Pinkberry after this, hell yes, I am.

"Your margins were clear," Dr. Esposito says, repeating Dr. Partridge's assessment, "and there is no standard of care for Stage 3 disease," he says, "let alone Stage 2c like you." Although I am not happy he's just let the cat out of the bag regarding my staging, the big picture sounds great to me. Not getting additional therapy suggests confidence in my cancer-free status. "There's no point in referring you to a clinical trial right now because you wouldn't qualify," he explains. "We do have one going on right now for a drug called ipilimumab, but it's for later-stage patients. If down the road your status changes, though, it's good to have you in our system." I thank him, buoyed by the notion I don't need him, and have forgotten the word "ipilimumab" by the time I get down into the lobby. He, meanwhile, will go on to write in his report of our meeting: "Her tumor showed features which increase her risk for recurrent disease, including depth of 8 mm, ulceration, and close deep surgical margin, given the scalp site. Disease can recur locally or can be metastatic." I'm glad I didn't know any of that then. I'm glad I didn't know what I was in for.

INTERLUDE

Immunotherapy 101

Immunotherapy is not like chemo or radiation. When it works (and unfortunately, it often doesn't) it coaxes your body's own defenses to attack disease—and then, astoundingly, to continue defending the body after treatment has ended.

In the past few years, as more of these treatments have been going into clinical trial and making headlines, the buzz has made them sound like the next big thing. The reality is that unlocking the mysteries that the immune system holds for cancer treatment has, for researchers, been a laborious—and often thankless—pursuit in a field that not too long ago was regarded by many as a dead-end fringe of science. Its moment has been a long time in coming. It all begins, as these stories so often do, with the personal.

In 1890, Elizabeth Dashiell was a teenage bone cancer patient at New York's Memorial Hospital—the same facility that would later become Sloan Kettering—and bone surgeon William B. Coley was her doctor. Her death just a few months after diagnosis moved Coley deeply, and spurred him to try to understand why some patients, like Dashiell, succumbed, while others survived. His research soon led him to observe that cancer patients who developed bacterial infections after surgery seemed to fare better than those who didn't—perhaps, he conjectured, because there was something in the bacteria that adversely affected tumors. In 1891, he began experimenting with injecting cancer patients with live bacterial cultures (Coley later developed a heat-killed version of his therapy)—and what became known as Coley's toxins produced durable regressions in some patients.

Coley continued to use his form of therapy on nearly a thousand patients for the following 40 years of his career. But with the rise of radiation and chemo—and the inconsistent patient response rate to his toxins—the treatment was eventually assigned "new drug" status by the FDA and essentially banned from use.

But the work of Coley and his colleagues was encouraging enough to keep the flame going. In 1953, with the help of a $2,000 grant from Nelson Rockefeller, Coley's daughter, Helen Coley Nauts, and her friend Oliver R. Grace founded the Cancer Research Institute—the first and still only nonprofit organization in the world dedicated solely to cancer immunotherapy.

"She really felt immunotherapy had been abandoned by the medical community prematurely," says Jill O'Donnell-Tormey, the institute's chief executive officer and director of scientific affairs, "because she tracked hundreds of patients that her father treated, and saw that many of them had benefits. You're probably talking less than 10 percent, but these people didn't die of cancer; they died of other things. Many years after. She was convinced it was because of Coley's toxins. As Lloyd Old, who was head of our scientific advisory council for 40 years, used to say to her, 'Helen, the science has to catch up to your father.' " And when Old, who was also the William E. Snee Chair of Cancer Immunology at Memorial Sloan Kettering, died in 2011, his New York Times *obituary called him "the patriarch and chief proponent of a nascent branch of cancer treatment known as immunology."*

Of course, if you or someone you care about has had cancer in the past several decades, you most likely didn't have the luxury of waiting for science to catch up. As a wise friend once put it to me, there's a difference between treating a patient and curing a disease. All these years, as doctors have continued to treat patients, researchers have continued persistently to try to cure disease.

That journey has been a challenging one. Nobody would suggest that protocols like chemo or radiation or surgery are easy, but the job they do on cancer cells is more straightforward. My friend Steve, who is both the most die-hard Burning Man veteran I know and a big smarty-pants head of research at a California biotech company, explains it like this: "Tumor cells are evasive. If you look across treatment, there are the cytotoxic drugs [like the ones used in chemo]—they kill cancer cells, but kill anything else in your body that's dividing rapidly. That's the traditional way of treating tumors." In contrast, the elegance of immunotherapy is its selectivity. When it works, the body recognizes and destroys the cancer, with little or no collateral damage.

But getting a handle on the human immune system has taken—and continues to take—a lot of time and a lot of trial and error. Modern immunotherapy's main forerunner is interleukin-2, an immune system treatment for patients with metastatic cancer that is infrequently used, sporadically effective, and famed mostly as the stuff they gave Izzie on Grey's Anatomy when she had Stage 4 melanoma. "It was one of the original cancer therapy drugs," says Steve. "It was used in kidney cancer and melanoma. It turned out that it didn't work very often—but in a rare number, patients were completely cured." As time passed, he says, "We got to understand better about the immune system and how cancer cells subvert it." The immune system is smart. It learns. It remembers. The challenge has been harnessing it, but we're getting there. It's not the typical scorched-earth policy to cancer treatment. It's an activation of the body's own incredible weaponry.

And now, after decades of research, immunology is finally having a moment. New drugs offer hope for patients with once near-unbeatable cancers. There have been breakthrough vaccines like Gardasil, which prevents human papillomavirus (HPV), the virus that can lead to *cervical cancer, and Provenge, to treat prostate cancer. There have been profoundly promising successes in what's called adoptive T cell therapy, a process by which a patient's T cells are collected, reengineered, and then reintroduced into the body to fight cancer.*

And then there is what I eventually got: monoclonal antibody therapy. Cancer ingeniously sabotages the brakes, or checkpoints, of the immune system. It suppresses the body's natural aggressive, take-no-prisoners response. But one way to get around it is to go in via what are called checkpoint inhibitors: therapies that essentially release those brakes. It begins by introducing man-made antibodies into the patient that then bind themselves to the killer T cells, releasing them to attack cancer like Pac-Man devouring pellets. It's an ingenious means of bypassing the dangerous signal that cancer sends to disrupt the immune system and allowing the body to do what it's supposed to do: kill those sonofabitch cancer cells—and only the cancer cells.

"Cancer is adaptable," says James Allison. "It's incredibly able to deal with change. Unless you take out that last cancer cell, it can come back. But step back 200 feet. What we know about the human immune system is that it's also designed to be adaptable. It's designed for this.*"*

CHAPTER 6

One in Three

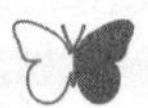

November 2010

The last time I saw my friend Carolyn was so long ago that Lucy was still a toddler in a stroller. But today we are together, eating lunch at an artsy bistro near an old movie theater and celebrating many things, including our forthcoming autumn birthdays, conveniently located just a few days apart. I find cancer has been an incredible motivator in my social life. "This place is great," she tells me. "I used to come here with Georgiana."

Georgiana was Carolyn's adventurous, outdoorsy workmate. She was in her 30s when life handed her a degenerative—and fatal—soft tissue disease. As we dive into our tomato soup and bread, Carolyn speaks lovingly of her comrade—of the swift diagnosis, of her slow, wrenching decline, and of her dry sense of humor. "Near the end," she recalls, "she thought I was spending too much time with her. She used to tell me, 'You know, I'm not going to be around much longer. You'd better start making some new friends.' "

"I think one of the most annoying things about having a terminal prognosis would be feeling like everybody is just waiting around for me to die," I say. "I wouldn't want people to look at me like, 'What are you still doing here?' "

"Oh, hi! I thought you were supposed to be dead weeks ago!" Carolyn laughs. Then she adds, quite sensibly, "I want something sparkly," and orders us two glasses of Prosecco.

"To your health," I say.

"To yours," she replies, and our glasses make a happy clink.

We spend the rest of the afternoon browsing pawnshops and thrift stores. "It's the photo albums that make me sad," she says, as we leaf together through a leather volume filled with images of Nixon-era hairstyles and casual smoking. "These people are probably all dead," I observe idly, "and now they're going to wind up in some idiot hipster's art project."

These ticket stubs and playbills and matchbooks, these graduation day photos and wedding invitations, they once meant everything to the person who lived them. Now they're just a curiosity on a table in a shop. Although my mementos may not someday appear underneath a jackalope and next to a set of Fonzie jelly jar glasses, in time all those letters and photo booth strips that added up to my life will be gone too. I understand that now. I'm here for a time, and then I'll be just a memory, like a photo of an unknown man with a wide collar and a Pall Mall dangling from his lips. Thank God that day isn't here yet.

When my birthday rolls around a few days later, I am the happiest to mark one more year on the planet than I have been since I turned 21—and back then I celebrated the milestone by drinking something with a worm in it. No matter what happens from here on in, I most likely have more time behind me than ahead. My head is changed, permanently damaged and weird, and currently still rebuilding itself and slathered in ointment. My free and unfettered pleasure of walking down the street on a sunny day has changed. My friendships have changed, and a few apparently have already evaporated altogether.

But I've had people I didn't think even remembered me tell me they love me. I got to hear the stuff most people don't get said about them until their funerals. I can still work. I can still run. I can still hug my family. I'm still here. I think I did get the best summer ever after all. It was the one that saved my life.

A few days after my birthday, exactly three months to the day after my diagnosis, it's 10 p.m. and I am uncharacteristically online, working on a story I have to file first thing in the morning. I give so much of my day to the Internet that I'm strict about avoiding it at night. Tonight, however, I have to be in front of the glowing screen, layering my notes into what I hope will become coherent sentences, when a distracting *bloop* tells me I have a new message. It's from Debbie, and it's addressed to me, Jill, Michele, and four other close friends. The subject is "My Lady Parts."

"Sorry for the big group email," it begins. "I had an appointment today with my new gynecologist, and he confirmed that I have ovarian cancer. I'm getting CT scans tomorrow to see if anything else shows up, and he's going to do a hysterectomy on Wednesday. I'm told to expect to be in the hospital three to five nights, and then have a four-week recovery. After that I'll get chemotherapy, the amount depending on what he sees during the surgery. Then I'll be all better and life will go on. The upside is he told me clear liquids include vodka. I like him."

I read the email three times in a row, hoping each time that this time, the words will be different.

Then I think, No you don't, cancer. Take me; I'm a jackass anyway. But you can't have Debbie. The person who, all those youthful Valentine's Days that I didn't have a valentine, not only always sent me one but signed it from Jan Brady's imaginary boyfriend, George

Glass. The person who responded to my diagnosis by making me a FUCK CANCER shirt. No.

I pick up the phone and hit the star marked "favorites." Debbie's husband, Mike, answers. I recognize the shell shock in his voice the moment he says, "Hi."

"I got the email. How's it going?" I ask, stupidly, helplessly.

"We're coping," he says. "It's not like we can do anything else. Here, let me get my wife."

He puts Debbie on the phone. The first thing she says is "I think I'm going to need my shirt back."

Welcome to the club, Debbie. One in three women will develop some form of cancer in their lives. Yet somehow this was a uniform I never imagined you'd have to wear.

She fills me in on more of the details of her situation, and how what she thought was a minor surgery for cysts escalated into a diagnosis and a fast track for surgery and chemo. She is shocked and pissed. Her arrival in this new place, like mine, has been abrupt and confusing. "We're all kind of stunned," she says. "I don't want to be Cancer Lady. I don't want to be the bald woman everybody feels bad for. This is not the plan. I'm supposed to get old."

I wish I could promise her it will all be okay. People do that—they confidently tell you it'll all be all right, and that's just bullshit. When we lived in Brooklyn, I had a friend named Anna. Anna was gorgeous and smart, as were her husband and two kids. She got breast cancer in her early 30s. She was already fit and healthy before the cancer, but after it, she went all in. She eliminated sugar, white flour, alcohol, and meat. She meditated and took supplements and juiced. The family left the city and moved upstate to the country for the fresh air and slower pace. Four years later, Anna died anyway. Because the inconvenient truth is that cancer sometimes just doesn't care how virtuous you are or how much you have to live for. Cancer is a dick like that.

So I don't feed Debbie useless lies. Instead I say, "I can't speak for the doctors, but here's what I can tell you. About a third of the people you know will step up and do great stuff for you because that's who they are and they would do it for anyone in trouble. A third of them will never get it together and cannot deal, and that's just how it is. The rest will do whatever they can, and they'll do it just because they love you, Debbie. We're the ones who love you. We love your guys too."

"It'll be okay," she says reassuringly. "You and I—we got married together, we had our babies together, and we're going to die together. When we're 90." Sounds like a plan.

The next day I go on Etsy and start plugging in words based solely on their history of amusing Debbie. It doesn't take too long to land on a subtle, organic cotton T-shirt emblazoned with a curlicue triangle and, in bold letters, the word MERKIN. I think that will do nicely.

It's an unseasonably warm evening one week later. My friend Stacey and I are perched at the bar at the Amsterdam Ale House, paying marginal attention to the ESPN blaring from the television. I'm wearing my new go-to uniform of loose, flowing clothing and a tightly tied scarf that conceals layers of gauze. "I know what you're thinking," I say as Stacey sizes me up. "Why is she out on a Friday night, and where are her eight identically dressed children?"

Stacey teaches yoga at my local studio, and like me, she's a theater nerd and mom. We have something else in common now too—cancer. Last year, she was diagnosed with the "good kind" of thyroid cancer. A small scar from her surgery sits near the hollow of her throat, like a pendant without a chain.

"You look great," she tells me. I get this a lot lately. Once I hit 40, I started assuming "You look great" came with a silent "for your age" at the end. Now I think there's an implied "for your cancer." Yet for one who's skated by on an incredibly lazy personal maintenance plan her entire life, I do look great. I've been eating right, sleeping great, and doing all the limited physical activity I can. Aside from the Pucci scarf covering the open, oozing sore where the malignant cancer was and the two tiny, probably unrelated little nodules on my lung that turned up on the CT scan I had a few weeks ago, I'm in the best shape of my life.

"You look great too. Your scar's faded so much since I first met you," I observe.

"Yeah, but I don't ever want it to go away completely," she says. "I want to remember, every time I look in the mirror. It reminds me what I survived." I'm still too newly brokenhearted over my head to agree with her, but I try to hope the scars will someday provide character. The bald spot? I'll tell people I got it in Desert Storm. The red rectangle on my thigh? Secret Russian mob tattoo. That clean little notch in my neck? Knife fight in Juárez.

It's becoming clear lately that I'm not the only scarred one around here. It's just that some wounds are more visible than others. The kids have begun to rechannel their anxiety about my illness into some straight-up surly, uncooperative behavior toward their still feeble mom. They leave a devastating trail of socks and squeezy yogurt wrappers everywhere, and I fully doubt they would bathe or wear shoes without elaborate and vaguely threatening reminders. Part of it is simply their ages—you don't get to be ten and six without routinely acting like hotel room–trashing rock stars, whacked out on Capri Sun. There is, I suppose, something encouragingly indomitable about the human spirit to be found in the solipsism of a child. She will only give so much of a crap about your oozing wounds or fear of mortality, and then she will expect you to provide her a peanut butter sandwich, no crust, and a glass of milk—and damned if taking care of her doesn't take you out of your own terrified, self-absorbed head.

Another part of this, though, is surely cancer-related acting out. This is Lucy's last year of elementary school, and thanks to New York's brutally ruthless and competitive public school system, we are already hip deep in a fall filled with the blood sport of tests and tours at middle schools all over the city. The kid would have been stressed enough without Cancer Mom to deal with. Throw in that monkey wrench, and she's been bumming out on the inconveniences my disease and recuperation have imposed on her and Bea. I've tried to be a trouper, but I still haven't been able to be the slumber party–hosting, bake sale–dominating champ of school years past. Subsequently, Lucy has been expertly playing the tween angst card, as only a daughter of a working, recovering-from-illness woman can.

This morning, I'm in the bedroom sorting through a mountain of laundry searching for two even vaguely matching socks when Lucy looks at the pile with angry disdain. "You're always going off somewhere and leaving us," she gripes.

"What do you mean?" I ask. "I haven't taken a trip since I did that reading in San Francisco, and that was almost two years ago."

"You're going to Costa Rica, aren't you?" she replies. So that's what this is about.

I wasn't much for sun and sand and jungle even before the melanoma thing. But when Jill and Michele sent out an email to a circle of friends back in April—long before my cancer diagnosis, well before I first felt that little bump on my head—to go in on a house and spend a ladies-only Thanksgiving week in a small Costa Rican surfing town, I decided before I'd finished reading it that I had to make it happen.

I knew the idea of gallivanting off to Central America for that most American and family-centric of holidays would raise a few eyebrows. I also knew, screw it; I don't get a lot of invitations to drink margaritas with a bunch of lesbians in Costa Rica. Jeff had been encouraging—exotic opportunities don't often come along, so if one person gets a chance to travel, the other always steps up to make it happen. What I couldn't have predicted was how the trip would come at an optimum moment for my firstborn to do some serious guilt-tripping.

"You're always gone," she repeats. "You were gone a long time for your surgery." I was gone one night.

I look at her, steaming there with resentment, and feel the urge to launch into another of our regular "No I'm not/Yes you are" standoffs. "Did you brush your teeth and comb your hair?" I instead reply, as I regard her tangled mass of snarls. We have exactly one minute to get out the door if we're not going to be late for school, though you wouldn't know it from the defiantly indifferent attitude of my progeny.

"No," she answers, like it's a wild idea. "You didn't tell me to."

"We do this every day. You know how to get ready for school."

"You're my mommy, you're supposed to tell me what to do," she snaps back.

"You're in the fifth grade and you're supposed to know what to do," I snarl, exasperated. "So brush your teeth and comb your hair." She stalks off, furious, and does the angriest bit of grooming I have ever witnessed.

As Lucy, Bea, and I walk in awkward silence to school, it dawns on me. This is not about Costa Rica, or tooth brushing, for that matter. I had surgery. I was zonked out recuperating for weeks. I couldn't even promise my children that I'd get better. I was gone. I frightened Lucy that I might get even more gone. She's not trying to make my life hard. She's finishing elementary school and leaving her friends in June. She just wants her mom to stick around to be the one to nag her. Because she's the kid and I'm her mom and that's important to her right now. Ohhhhh. I cannot imagine how scary it was for her when I got sick, and she—the responsible, mature, dutiful daughter, all of ten years old—felt the weight of all that.

"Listen, I didn't get it before but I do now," I say. "I hear you when you say you need my help. I'm here to take care of you, okay? I'm always Mom and I will always take care of you. I don't want to fight."

"Me neither," she says.

"Were you worried," I ask, "when I was sick?"

"Duh, Mom," Lucy answers. "I was afraid you were going to die."

I kiss both my little girls goodbye. Although I'm sure I'm giving my daughters plenty of material for their future shrinks every day, I'm still around to screw them up. Go ahead and piss me off, kids. Tell me I drive you crazy and that I'm so mean. You have no idea how important it is to me that you're just the little girls with the crazy-making mean mom. Because it's a whole lot better than being the ones with the dead mom.

CHAPTER 7

Christmas Is Over

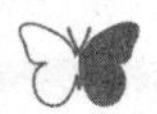

Thanksgiving 2010

Even the main street of Mal País is not paved. It's basically the only street—a bumpy strip dotted with hostels, surf shops, and casual restaurants where patrons sip Imperial beer and fruit smoothies and stray dogs lazily assert their right-of-way by parking in our path.

The heavy humidity that's been diligently frizzing what's left of my hair since we landed had not abated in the least when we walked into the house. In fact, it had seemed damper inside, with a mildewed aroma permeating the air. Aside from the native moistness, however, the place is stunning: high ceilings, full kitchen, tranquil swimming pool and patio, and big rooms with hammocks on their private decks. Jill, Michele, and I had dropped off our bags when we got in, and then, famished, walked down the road to the first friendly-looking joint we could find while the rest of our friends trickled in back at the house.

We are eating lunch at an open-air establishment with a dirt floor and rustic roof to keep out the rain. I am having the *casado*—the house meal—a plate of chicken, rice, and beans. It's cheap and simple and so delicious I could weep. "Everything here is so fresh," Jill says. "The last time I was here I felt like I'd gone through detox by the time we left." I see my plan for the week unfolding before me already. No painkillers or weird CT scan dyes running through my veins. None of NYC's abundance of grime and noise and hassle. Just the chance to feel cleaner and clearer and lighter of heart.

"Have you talked to Debbie?" I ask Jill. Her surgery was just two days ago, and considerably more invasive than mine. Her cancer was staged at 2c, and she's starting chemo in January.

"I have," she says. "She's wiped out but she sounds good. She just wants to be well enough to enjoy Thanksgiving."

I'm still getting the hang of my post-melanoma identity, and of being the person who travels with a small supply of Silvadene and a dorky purple headscarf, of being the yogi who's not going to attempt a headstand. I'm also determined, however, this new person is never going to put off another damn thing—like going for sunrise walks by the Pacific or spending time with friends I love. During the heat of the day, while my friends are happily surfing and sunbathing, I prefer to feel the spray of the ocean and watch monkeys leap around the trees from the safety of a shady yoga class on a pergola right out on the beach. The teacher is an impossibly beautiful French woman with a hypnotically lilting accent. I am immediately hooked.

Despite my best efforts at being 100 percent half-assed, there is something new about my practice here that moves me. The awareness that being in a different place brings. The incessant chatter inside my head quieted down a few notches. The worrying that I'm doing something wrong gone, replaced with a sense of pliancy and suppleness. Just soft inhalations and exhalations, my breathing so much smoother and easier than my usual tense, shallow respiration. I stretch forward, unwinding my too often too tight limbs toward each other.

I sink deeply and wrap my hands around my feet, and hands and feet delight in meeting each other.

"How was the class?" Jill asks as I languidly stroll in to the house after my session.

"Good," I reply. "Nothing too strenuous. Lots of stretching. No funny business."

"Ah," she says, "tourist yoga."

"Exactly," I say, as I crack open an Imperial. I may not be on the fast track to enlightenment with my remedial hatha and beer plan, but it's my vacation-based spiritual path and I'll drink my way down it if I want to.

From then on, the days work out brilliantly. Yoga. Watermelon margarita that tastes like summer crossed with tequila and burying myself in a book at the bar, followed by deep tissue massage. I stroll over to the cabana, undress, and slip under a vibrant pareu. The ocean breeze blowing in is soft and salty. If I opened my eyes, I could see the sunlight streaming in. I choose instead to close them and let the masseuse knead me until I'm limp. She smooths lavender-scented potions into my calves; she slides her hands down my back and the curve of my spine. I roll lazily over and she places a hand softly over my heart. Although I know now that my body can be a vicious bitch, I am still proud of what it can also be. It can grow a baby. It can do a backbend. It can entwine with a lover. It's regenerating a scalp right now. Even starfish and earthworms would be impressed.

Each day of the week, I dutifully apply sunscreen, a process that is extensive and needs to be repeated constantly. Each day I do it more lovingly, relearning the terrain of my body with each application. I am so pissed at it for turning my own cells against me, but I'm impressed at how responsive it is. I want to be friends with my flesh from here on in: the paleness, the moles, the laugh lines, the calluses on my feet, the allergic reactions to shellfish, the blushes at inopportune situations, and then—the kicker—the way it tried to kill me. My body is not the enemy. It is a force to be reckoned with. Of all the things I can give thanks for this faraway Thanksgiving, this year, I'm going to start with that.

December 25, 2010

Jeff's folks have come over to exchange Christmas gifts and share a humble dinner of roast chicken and gingerbread. It's a quiet, restful day, especially because a third of the assembly has been dealing with cancer recently. Dad is sitting by the tree, smiling. He's lost a few pounds this time around on the chemo, but it looks good on him. He is now fully immersed in his regimen. He goes in on Mondays for treatment and then back on Tuesdays for a refill, one week on and one week off. In the off weeks he can still get around and rehearse with the church choir. In the on weeks he's wiped out. The girls know he cannot play with them as much, but they're patient with him. Next month he and Mom are going to Florida, and they're both eager for the break.

"The tree is beautiful," Dad observes to me as we sit amid the detritus of the morning's unwrapping frenzy. "Don't you find that everything seems more beautiful now? I'm so emotional. We went to Alvin Ailey a few nights ago and I cried the whole performance." He gives a chuckle, embarrassed by his candor.

I nod in assent. "How's the treatment going?" I ask. "You look great." I cannot help adding a silent "for your cancer" in my head.

"I feel good," he says. "I hope it's working. I just don't like it when the doctor starts talking to me about 'my' cancer. I don't want to call it that. It's not me. I just want it out of there."

Dad is fundamentally combative and rarely takes well to disagreement, so I am unsurprised by his adversarial approach. Though I know I'm risking putting myself on the receiving end of his eternal eagerness for a debate, I nonetheless must beg to differ. "Well, my cancer is my cancer," I say. "It's my body, it's my cells. I feel like I have to be peaceful toward it. I don't want to rile it up. Does that sound crazy?"

"We all find our own way," he answers gently.

Later, as he and Mom pile on their coats and gather up their presents, Dad gazes around the living room wistfully. "I guess Christmas is really over," he sighs. A wave of sadness engulfs us all. Jeff and I flick a glance toward each other, and I know what we're both thinking. Dad is already missing this Christmas because he's wondering if he will see the next one. Sickness has a way of forcing you to confront mortality in ways you never imagined. It's not just "Oh, la di dah, I wonder if I have soul." It's "What if my last birthday was my last birthday?" It's "What if there are no more Christmases?" I watch Dad take one more look back toward us as he and Mom get in the elevator with their presents. He will never walk through our door again.

CHAPTER 8

Bad Hair Day

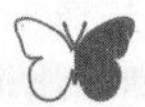

January 2011

I guess this is a new tradition, starting the year holding my breath in a machine. It's been three months since my last set of CT scans, so I get to kick off 2011 with another. Though Dr. Partridge tells me the two little spots are still detectable on my lung, the news is good. My medical report notes that they're "unchanged," and there are "no new nodules." It feels like an auspicious portent, a new beginning, after a year of such drastic tumult.

We mark the girls' joint birthday with two kinds of celebration, two kinds of cake, and me having only one small nervous breakdown during the slumber party. The weekend after, we go out to the folks' house for considerably more sedate festivities. Mom and Dad take us all out for a special lunch at their favorite local restaurant, where Dad is treated like a visiting dignitary by the staff, who haven't seen him as much lately since the chemo started again. He looks thrilled to be back, like old times.

"I'm doing very well," he tells our waiter. "Barbara and I are going to Florida soon. It'll be nice to get away from the cold." After our meal, he detours us to the bookstore on the way home, where he tells the kids to pick a treat. Lucy agonizes over a stack of potential novels she wants, but Bea has other plans. She is holding a small stuffed unicorn and asking imploringly, "Does it have to be a book?"

"No," Dad says, laughing. "It doesn't have to be a book." It is a good weekend.

Two weeks later, Jeff goes to White Plains again to attend a Saturday afternoon party with his parents, while the girls and I stay behind to catch up on homework and Sunday school. It is not a good weekend.

A few days ago, Dad woke up in the morning saying his feet hurt. He's developed neuropathy, seemingly overnight. It's a fairly common side effect of some forms of chemo—a nerve pain that usually occurs in the hands and feet. And it's serious business—it can make just taking a few steps agony. His feet have also swollen, and on this January day, he has to go to the party in slippers that have been cut open to accommodate his suddenly overinflated condition. A trip across the living room from his chair to the couch takes several minutes and requires both Jeff's and Jeff's mother's assistance. He and Mom have reluctantly and disappointedly canceled their trip to Florida, and his doctors have suspended his chemo.

February 2011

When Jeff goes out again to Westchester for another weekend social event—his minister parents have a lot of friends—Dad seems vastly improved. He's back on the chemo, and his physical therapist is talking about going for walks outside soon. On Sunday, Jeff goes to church with him, and though Dad walks with a cane, he's walking nonetheless. He tells the pastor, "I'll be singing in the choir by Easter." At the coffee hour afterward he chats with his old friends, including a woman who's a fellow cancer patient, and they talk about how they both believe in and feel the presence of angels in their lives.

"The old man knows how to rally," Jeff tells us when he comes home for dinner Sunday night.

Debbie, meanwhile, is now three months past surgery and healing well. There was a valentine in the mailbox last week from her. It was not, as she used to send when we were single, from my imaginary boyfriend, George Glass. It was instead a homemade collage of classic friends from history—Thelma and Louise, Bart and Milhouse, Laverne and Shirley, SpongeBob and Patrick, Charlotte and Wilbur, all the girls from *Facts of Life*. Inside it read, "I love you, man."

Over my lunch break, I call her up to check in on her and to oh so casually ask, "How goes the cancer?"

"Not bad," she replies. "After the hysterectomy, my doctor told me not to have sex or do any sports for a few weeks," she tells me, laughing, "and I said, 'No problem, lady.' " She started her chemo a few weeks ago. "I look like a Harry Potter villain," she says. "Tim calls me Voldemom. At first, nothing was happening and I thought maybe I'd get off easy. Then one day in the shower it all kicked in. Now I can yank out fistfuls of hair at a time. It's great for freaking out the kids. All these years, I was plucking and shaving. Now? Smoother than I ever dreamed."

"Don't think of it as losing your hair," I say. "Think of it as a full-body Brazilian." Then I deploy an old college game. "Would you rather," I begin, "lose all your hair all over your body for six months, or lose five centimeters of hair off your head forever?"

"That's a trick question," she replies. "Because the answer is: You don't get to decide." *Ding ding ding,* give that lady the prize.

Always stealthily subversive, Debbie has become newly ferocious of late. She's changed her Facebook profile picture to a lollipop-brandishing image of Kojak. She posts pictures of herself, bald and wearing a tiny, glittery cowboy hat.

She has been talking lately to a therapist, referred by her oncologist as part of her hospital's cancer care. I've known Debbie for more than 20 years, and I have barely ever heard her talk about her feelings. That's what I like about her. No drama. But I'm hopeful about her exploring this course as part of her treatment. There's nothing like a life-threatening illness to saddle a person with an abundance of new emotions just screaming to get out.

Her therapist, however, seems like a poor fit. Debbie tells me, "She keeps asking, 'Why do you come in here smiling? Why are you laughing and making jokes? I'm worried you're not dealing with this.' I'm thinking, *Bitch, you're 30 and you don't have kids. Don't tell me how I'm supposed to feel. You have no idea how I'm holding it together.*"

"Don't take this the wrong way," I tell her, "but she sounds like a moron. She can't handle that you don't fit the mold of cancer patient she read about in some book."

"When I first came in," she says, "she gave me a questionnaire, and all the questions were like, 'Do you feel hopeless? Do you feel like harming yourself?' I'm not depressed, I have cancer. Where's the part on the form about wanting to get better?"

"Seems like your shrink is very disappointed when you're not all sad and tragic," I say. "She has no clue. She doesn't know how much it matters to be able to smile. I'm cleaning my head with a vagina pick. I get head enemas now, Deb. Am I supposed to cry about that?"

"Well," she replies, "I wouldn't exactly be happy about it either."

"I'm just over hearing people without cancer tell those of us who've experienced it how we're supposed to do it," I say. "Like there's always got to be a struggle or a fight, and it's supposed to be courageous. You know what? Bite me."

"God, I can't stand the 'battling' talk. I'm just trying to live my life. Don't assume I'm a warrior because I got sick. I'm not suiting up for D-Day," Debbie says, adding, "It's the word 'lost' that really gets me. Lost a battle. How do you win?"

"I didn't get that memo," I reply. "Is it when you make it a year? Five years? Live forever? Do people who get hit by cars lose a battle with traffic? It's like that Onion headline I love: 'World Death Rate Holding Steady at 100 Percent.' "

Yet when I think about our conversation later that day, I wonder if I shouldn't be so hard on the language of battle. How else, after all, could I possibly describe what's going on with my hair? Now that the wound has mostly closed and is less sticky, I don't need gauze over it anymore, and don't have to worry about stray hairs getting stuck in my scabs. On the downside, that circle on the top of my head will forevermore be bald, and is for the immediate future underneath a protective layer of A+D ointment. My head resembles a monk's tonsure and smells like a baby's ass. I will always have to style it against the natural part, scraping the handle of a comb down my scalp and moving it to the wrong side, to at least partially cover the bald spot. I'm also still not yet allowed to color it—I have to put up with conspicuous roots that make me look like the cover girl for *Meth Head Monthly* a few more weeks.

I do what I can to cover my scar, so the sun won't burn more cancer around the part of my scalp the doctors removed—and also because I don't want my freakishness to make people uncomfortable. And by people, I mostly mean my own children. I hate that the girls still get squicked when they catch a glimpse of my pate. When a bit of newly formed scalp peeps through when we're in public, Bea tugs on my arm and whispers, "Mom. Your bald spot," and then I quickly swoop my hair to the side, like Donald Trump caught in an updraft. I don't want to embarrass her.

This sick person's head I now possess represents everything I've lost, everything I've become. I am a misread name on a chart, a statistic to be beaten or to become. I am a tangled mess of dark roots and gray growth and faded-out Feria by L'Oréal. I don't want to be this person, any more than Debbie wants to be Voldemom. So maybe there's redemption to be found in the Rite Aid.

Tonight, the girls and I stand together in the bathroom. We take turns running long, plum-colored temporary streaks through our hair and fiddling with brightly colored flowered barrettes. The girls drag their wands through their locks with enviable carelessness; I cautiously steer clear of my roots around my wound. It's not just vanity that brings us here to the mirror now. It's not just play, either. It's the desire that streak by streak, we can claim back some of the terrain that cancer took away.

CHAPTER 9

Spring Breakdown

March 2011

"Do you want to go to Rocky Mountain National Park today?" Julie asks. "It's pretty spectacular." I've only ever seen the Rockies from the windows of airplanes, and then only when seated on the more advantageous side of the plane. Yes, please, I would very much like to see the Rockies for the first time, for real, and I'm plenty stoked to have a good friend who invited me to come out so she could show them to me.

Back home, Lucy has a classmate's long-anticipated sleepover birthday party lined up for this weekend, and Jeff and Bea have planned some special one-on-one father-daughter time. I, meanwhile, am drinking freshly ground, super-dark, rich coffee and eating granola so delicious it might just ruin me, with one of the healthiest people I've ever met. We met when we both lived in San Francisco, but she's a perfect fit for Boulder. Julie is a divorced mom who skis, runs, bikes, eats right, and wears sunscreen. She glows with vibrant energy. But she's not invulnerable.

More than ten years ago, Julie was diagnosed with a melanoma on her abdomen and had surgery to remove it. "It still sometimes hits me how serious it was," she says as her cat mewls at imaginary prey at the back door. "I was so young—29. So now I'm on it—anything looks different, I go to the doctor right away." She gets regular skin checks and takes care of herself. Her only health issue now is that she takes antidepressants and sees a shrink. Diligence isn't her problem. Insurance is.

After she left her last job, Julie was paying into COBRA and wanted to switch to a plan that would cover her and her kids. Now, because of health care reform requiring that kids be approved for coverage, she tells me that some insurers have stopped writing plans for them. Rather than cover children, they're basically pretending they don't exist.

"Insurance is a gamble. If you buy car insurance, they're gambling that you won't get in an accident. Health isn't a gamble," she says. "Everybody, at some point, gets sick. Everybody has to go to the doctor."

Like a whole lot of us, Julie has been given plenty of reasons to feel flummoxed and exasperated by the health care system. "I got an MRI last year because of a knee injury and the bill was $800," she recalls. "My brother-in-law had to have one for a kidney stone when he was traveling in Vietnam, and you know how much it cost? Eight dollars. It was the same exact machine. Why don't we talk about the drug companies charging exorbitant amounts for pills, saying they have to, when they're spending millions to lobby before Congress and take out ads on prime-time television?" She has a thoroughly valid point. The Center for Public Integrity says that in 2007 alone, the pharmaceutical industry spent $168 million on lobbying.

"I went to an insurance broker," Julie continues, "and he steered me to a plan. I had to fill out paperwork on every doctor visit, every prescription, for my kids and me over the last five years. They called me and made me talk through everything, the reasons behind every visit. In the end, they told me they turned us down because I'm on

Cymbalta. It's ridiculous. I'm trying to take care of myself. Would they rather I get gastrointestinal problems or heart disease because of untreated depression?"

"They've got to have considered that too," I say. "Why do you think they wouldn't cover you?"

"I guess because I'm probably a lifer," she says. "They start adding up my pills and my psych visits. They look at me and they just see someone who needs maintenance." Yet I see in her someone who couldn't have her act more together—conscientious and fit—the type of person least likely to be a drain on the system.

After breakfast, as promised, Julie drives us up steep, winding roads where the snows are melting in the early March sun, but the trees are still bare. The day is flawlessly bright, and the mountains—well, they go on forever. "Pretty breathtaking" is the understatement of the year. When we get out of the car at a particularly awe-inspiring view, Julie has a question for me.

"How are you doing?" she asks. "The altitude starts to get to some people around here."

"I hadn't even thought about that," I say, happily surprised. I've never been in the mountains, any mountains, anywhere. How pleasant to discover, at this late stage in my life, a talent—I can take altitude like a champ.

"How are you doing, everything else–wise?" she asks cautiously.

"I'm fine," I say. It's been almost six months since my diagnosis. "My head's all closed up and I can color my hair again. They found a few spots on my lung when I went for my scans last fall, but they could be from anything. I grew up in New Jersey. I was living downwind of the Twin Towers on 9/11. I can't believe I don't have the respiratory system of a Welsh coal miner." Then I stop and think what a contrast my good fortune makes lately. "It's the men in my life who aren't doing so well," I tell her. "Jeff's dad's got colon cancer and now, because of the neuropathy, they don't know how long he can continue the chemo. I think it's going to be a miracle if he makes it out of this year alive."

"Does Jeff know that?" she asks.

"I don't believe he's entirely ready to," I say. "Sometimes he'll say that maybe we won't all be together for Thanksgiving. Dad's old, he's sick, but that's Jeff's family. Even with everything that's happened with Dad and Debbie and with me, it's still all abstract to him. The only person he's ever had die was his grandmother, and she was 92." I, on the other hand, feel more certain that we are in for heartbreaking changes. I just don't know how soon.

The next morning, Sunday, I am dashing through the Minneapolis–St. Paul airport, trying to make my connecting flight home. As I am shuttling between terminals, I feel a buzz in my pocket that indicates new voice mail. The ID says Jeff—but the voice on the message is Lucy's.

"Hi, Mommy," she says. "Can you call us as soon as you can?" My stomach instinctively drops. I move my carry-on bag over to my opposite shoulder as I frantically hit the "return call" button. It rings forever before Jeff picks up.

"Everything is all okay," he says, and the measured, halting sound of his voice plainly tells me it isn't. "It looks like Lucy had a reaction to the antibiotics." A few days ago, she'd been fighting off an ear infection. The pediatrician had prescribed a mild course of penicillin, and she was doing fine. "Yesterday she woke up covered in hives," he says. "Then last night we were on the way to Abby's slumber party, and she fainted."

"She what?" I reply, a little too loudly.

"Well, fortunately, she had her pillow with her, so she landed on that," he reassures, and I cannot resist smiling at the absurdity of the image. "She said she didn't feel well, and then she just crashed. We took her to the emergency room, and we had to wait around forever, but she's completely okay. It just shook her up. We didn't want to call you last night because we got back so late."

She's okay, I tell myself. In a few hours I'll be home. She's okay.

"There's something else," Jeff continues. "Dad's in the hospital. He and Mom went out to dinner Friday, and ever since he's been throwing up a lot. They thought it best to admit him."

"Well, with cancer they just need to be careful," I say. My brain is buzzing. Two hospital trips in the last 12 hours and I'm hundreds of miles away. I've never felt so helpless. The funny part is, I'd be just as helpless if I were home. I couldn't stop Dad or Lucy from getting sick. But I would be there. You're supposed to be there when it hits the fan.

"Just hang on," I tell him. "I'll be home soon."

On the tarmac, icy flecks begin to flutter down as I pop a Biscoff I squirreled away from the flight into my mouth. This day has already gone totally to hell, so I'm not in the least surprised when, before the last bit of cookie has melted on my tongue, I hear the announcement that my flight—along with the next several after it—has been canceled. By the time I finally do make it back to my own home, it's the early hours of Monday morning.

When I walk in the door at last, the first thing I do is the first thing I always do when I get in late. I peek in on the girls and their dreaming forms. Sometimes, when I look at them, I see the babies they once were, all flushed and milk drunk in my arms, their chubby hands curled around my finger. I remember them pulling up to standing in the crib, then plopping down on unsteady legs with surprised giggles. Other times, I look at them and see two young women, a bride and her maid of honor at a wedding, or two grubby travelers throwing down backpacks in the hall after a month hiking Central America together. I want to be there, I think, as I watch them from the doorway, for all of it.

When Lucy wakes up in the morning, she is still ravaged with hives. Bea looks decidedly off too, and I'm not exactly feeling like a million bucks either. So I keep both the kids home from school and take another day off from work and haul us over to the pediatrician. The doctor hooks Lucy up with a different antibiotic, and then casts an inscrutable look at Bea and me. She calls for her nurse. "Let's do a throat culture on these guys," she says, pointing to us. A few minutes later, she returns with the verdict. "Yep," she announces to my younger offspring and me, "it's strep." Seven days in, and March is already a hellscape.

Over bowls of pumpkin soup at dinner that night, Jeff updates the whole family on Dad's condition as diplomatically and nonscarily as he can. He needs to be observed so the doctors can determine if his vomiting and diarrhea are reactions to the chemo, or if it's the cancer. They've stopped the chemo again for now. "I spoke to Mom, and she suggested I go to see him," Jeff reports. "Sounds like he's going to be there a little while longer. I thought it'd be good for me to spend a few days out there and help her out, and commute into work from White Plains."

"Of course," I say.

"Lucy and I were talking yesterday," Jeff adds. "While I'm at Mom's, she wants to do your head."

Caring for my head is a chore—and a ritual that has become a daily act of devotion on Jeff's part. I knew him for 20 years before I got cancer. I knew him as a friend, a husband, a father, an ex. But I don't think either of us ever knew exactly what he had in him until he assumed the role of Chief Bandage Changer and Blood Cleaner. He's amazing at it. Half a year after surgery, my head still hurts. It's still scabby and sore and taut and shiny, and it aches and pulls as each new layer of flesh comes in. Jeff tends my head on a nightly basis with a squirt from the enema bottle, a gentle wipe of gauze, and a layer of ointment applied with a tongue depressor. It's hard for me to manage the job myself; when Jeff and I are apart, I have to rely on a hand mirror and my poor spatial reasoning to get it even close to right. Just from the past few days away in Colorado, the scar has grown all cracked and tight, and my cowlick is going crazy with all the A+D haphazardly smeared into it.

"I can handle it," Lucy chimes in. "I've watched Daddy take care of you every night. It's not that hard."

But one Scalp Caretaker per household is enough. My firstborn may still be a nightmare about putting her clothes in the hamper, but she is helpful and kind. She is also 11 and she should not have to clean up her mother's cancer surgery site. She's already done enough growing up for one year. Only a few months ago, we had that big fight because she was demanding that I take care of her. That was rough. Now she's insisting she can take care of me. This is rougher.

"I know you can handle it," I tell her, "but I don't want you to." She looks hurt, like I'm letting her down. "It's not that you wouldn't be great," I explain. "It's just this—I'm Mom. My job is to take care of you, not the other way around, remember? It's just for a few days. We'll all be okay. We'll all be back together soon." That's what I tell myself as Jeff packs an overnight bag and a few clothes and then leaves for the commuter train to White Plains. That's what I tell myself as the elevator door closes in front of him.

When I talk to Jeff later the next day, he's in good spirits. "I'm glad I came out," he says. "I think it was important for Mom. The old man's got spunk, I'll tell you that. They came by today with some Do Not Resuscitate forms and he told them, 'Not so fast!' "

"I'm not dead yet!" I say. "I feel happy!"

"He said to me, 'I told the doctors to do everything possible to keep me around. I'll be back in the church choir again in no time.' "

"And picking fights," I add.

"He says he just wants to see the spring," Jeff tells me. "Dad loves the spring." It's only three weeks away.

Sure enough, by the end of the week, Dad does indeed seem to be rallying. When I speak to him on the phone, his voice is hoarse but clear. "What's going on?" I ask.

"Well, it's not the vacation I'd planned," he deadpans. "But they're letting me try some solid food again, and that's going well."

"You get your rest and feel better soon," I say. "The girls have been asking when they can paint with Grandpa again."

I get off the phone more hopeful and clearheaded than I've felt in days. Dad's on the upswing, and the kids and I are likewise gratefully coming out of the fog of our respective ailments.

A few days later, Jeff calls with more encouraging news about Dad. "I'm not sure I understood correctly," he says, "but it sounds like the doctors think they can get him into some kind of cancer rehab place and on a different treatment. I don't know if it's new drugs or just a different kind of chemo."

"That's fantastic," I say, relieved. They'll deal with the neuropathy, and they'll get the chemo right, and Jeff will come home, and it'll be better. Not perfect, but better.

But that afternoon, it's all taken yet another turn. When I pick up Bea at school, her teacher tells me, in her gentle, progressive school way, "This was a hard day for her." This morning she'd told the teacher that she didn't feel good and sat out most of the day's activities, sobbing that she missed Daddy. Then it gets worse.

I'm almost finished walking the kids home from school through the bleak March chill, just outside our building, when Jeff calls. "We had a talk with the doctors today. They're moving Dad into hospice," he says. "The doctor actually said to me this morning, 'It's curtains.' "

"Whoa" is all I can muster, and I stop dead in my tracks. "Does he understand? How did he take it?"

The girls look at me with fear and I give an unconvincing wave of my hand, as if to signify it's not a big deal, and they accommodatingly run off down the street to give me a little privacy.

"He's in and out a lot," he explains. "So when the doctor told him, 'You may be here a week, a month, but you're not going to be able to go home,' he said, 'Well, that's a shock,' and then he fell asleep for a while. When he woke up, the first thing he told us was 'I guess I have to strengthen my faith.' Then he signed the Do Not Resuscitate."

He and his mom also have had to run defense—a few of Dad's well-meaning friends have been calling, trying to visit, trying to rouse him out of this late-stage cancer thing. "His friend Bob came by and told him he could beat this and come home," says Jeff. "That was a disaster." Dad was a wreck the rest of the afternoon, doubting the wisdom of his signing the DNR and questioning whether the doctors could do more.

"How are you?" I ask.

"Your whole life, you have your parents," he says. "I don't know how to not have them." I've spent much of my life not having my mother and father, in one way or another. Their absence has defined me in ways big and small. Like how I will never fully understand what Jeff is going through now. His grief is a privilege I'll never have.

"I'm going to get some dinner with Mom," he says. "Then I'm going back to the hospital to be with Dad, for however long it takes. I don't know how I'm going to do it, but I swear, I'm going to get through this month and I'm going to bury my father."

"Whether he's dead or not," I reply.

A puff of laughter escapes from the other end of the phone. "And that's why you're the woman for me," he says.

On the way to school the next morning, Lucy is muttering a poem to herself. "I'm nobody," she says. "Who are you?"

"Nobody too," I say. Lucy's going through a thing lately where she's fascinated with poetry. She scribbles haikus in her journals, and sometimes, she unconsciously marks meter with her fingertips as she talks. She's got an ear for it I've never mastered. Yet this morning, I cannot help remembering my own schoolgirl memorizations of Dickinson, and how wrong that Belle of Amherst turned out to be, about a lot of things. I'm not nobody, and death does not kindly stop for anybody. It barges in, not waiting a turn. It doesn't give a damn if you have your own stuff going on, or if one of your best friends does.

But Lucy, her romantic soul bubbling with verse, continues. "Do not go gentle into that good night. Rage, rage against the dying of the light." She halts to think about it. "Do you know that one?"

"Yes," I say. "I do."

"What's it mean?"

"It's about a man whose father is dying," I tell her. "The son doesn't want him to go. He wants him to fight."

Jeff harbors no such Dylan Thomas–like fury. Instead, whenever I speak to him, he pings between a merciful impatience for Dad's suffering to be over and an agonizing longing to keep just one more day, one more hour. There's no more to be done but wait. These days are just about comfort and grace, two of life's more elusive pleasures. Dad cannot even have solid food anymore. But he will not go sugar-free into that good night.

The next day Jeff calls me from a party supply store somewhere on Mamaroneck Avenue. This morning, when he and his mother had gone to see Dad, the nurse had warned them he'd pulled out his tubes during the night. There was blood everywhere. "I have found my purpose," he now says, sounding happier than I've heard him all month. "My dad wants lemon lollipops. I'll be goddamned if he's going to die without them." Jeff, the only child, the Little Emperor of his family. Ever the star, ever the one taken care of. This year, his father and I have given him the chance to become something new. The chance to be the one to take care of. To be the one with the lemon lollipops.

"He keeps saying he's sorry he's putting us through this," Jeff says. "He was asking this afternoon, 'Why doesn't God take me? I'm ready.' He apologized to me for taking so long." The only thing worse than feeling like you're disappointing people by dying has got to be feeling like you're disappointing people by remaining alive.

While Jeff keeps vigil at his father's bedside, the girls and I struggle through the day-to-day, the stuff of life that never relents even when you're otherwise in chaos. Lucy still has interviews and tests at the desirable public middle schools. There is Sunday school and the after-school art program, and there are bills to be paid and deadlines to be met. Yet we grasp for grace in our own ways. We find it in all sorts of random moments, clinging to each other for loving warmth this cold, strange month. It's there in the nights we pop in a movie and have quesadillas on a picnic blanket for dinner, or in quiet afternoons at the library. I cannot have all their memories of March be sad ones. I want my daughters to look back someday and recall the tender ones as well.

March 17, 2011

I am not my most pulled together this particular St. Patrick's Day. I had tried this morning to drop by Time Warner Cable on the way to the train station to replace our cable box, but the office was closed. I am consequently about to bring a large, broken piece of television equipment to my father-in-law's deathbed.

Jeff is bleary-eyed, unshaven, and he needs a haircut. His shirt looks like it's been slept in, and I swear he's grown a few new gray hairs in just the past week. Yet when I see him waiting for me at the Tarrytown train station, my heart melts. There's a melancholy maturity to him, an indefinable substance. I have never before felt more sure that this disheveled, rumpled mess is the man I love.

He throws his arms around me, and then pulls away quickly, embarrassed. "I'm kind of gross," he says. "I smell like hospital." He does. There's an unforgettably strange aroma on him, a scent both antiseptic and primal, like medicine and disease.

"I want you to prepare yourself," Jeff says as we drive toward the hospice. "Dad doesn't look like Dad."

"It's okay," I tell him. I am brazenly confident this particular part should be a snap. After all, I've watched enough people prepare themselves for me. Ever since my surgery, every time another friend sees me for the first time, I watch that flicker of self-steeling on their faces, that tight, frozen, Academy Awards nominee whose name has just not been called look. I have seen that look enough to know how to mimic it, that poker face of bad news.

Of course, in my case, it's usually followed by a subtle sigh of relief. I am, aside from the head scar that still needs care, in good health. I tend not to run at my loved ones like a bull, my angry, hot pink wound charging headlong at them. I wear concealing hats and fanciful barrettes and sport a clever comb-over. I try to put people at ease, to not make them feel they're in the company of a freak. Scars and all, I'm not so hard to look at. I'm not in the final stages of disease. Dad is.

It takes five minutes to drive to the hospice, every moment of which is spent with Jeff chattering nervously all the way. In just two weeks at Dad's bedside, he's dropped out of the rhythm of regular life. He cannot speak of sports scores or *American Idol* results or Beltway politics or vacation plans. All he knows right now are morphine drips and interrupted sleeps. All he knows is that his father is dying.

By the time I walk into the room, my confidence has evaporated and I am shaky with the gut-twisting knowledge that this is the last time I will ever be with Dad. Mom, who has been sitting silently by the window, looks up and rises to give me a hug. We wrap arms around each other in a big squeeze. "It's good to see you," she says.

"You too," I agree, and it is. There is good in the sad stuff. There is good in the pain. I wonder why I never knew that before.

At the foot of the bed, a TV is set to peaceful scenes of flowers and mountain streams and sunsets. Very *Soylent Green*. "Please," I whisper to Jeff, "when it's my time, just give me a continuous loop of C-Span *Book TV,* so you can tell people I was literally bored to death."

The hale, chubby Dad I sat with at lunch and shared birthday cake with in January is gone. This man is considerably thinner. His chin is dotted with stubble, and his flesh is thickly mottled with dark purple lesions. A tube coming out of his nose helps him breathe, and another one in his abdomen drains swampy, green-brown fluid from his stomach into a pitcher in a steady flow. It's called ascites, but I think "sludge" says it all. This is what late-stage cancer looks like. It's rotting him before my eyes. It scares me damn near out of my mind. I hadn't been prepared for this after all.

"Hey there," I say softly, as I move toward the bed.

He acknowledges my entrance with a faint nod and weakly extends his hand. I take it gently, my fingers caressing his papery flesh. "Can I go now?" he whispers. "I'm ready to go." He seems so serene.

I pat his hand lovingly. "Soon," I say. "We're all right here with you."

"I have to go," he says again. What beautiful acceptance, I think. What calm dignity. Then he adds, "I have to go pee." Oh.

"When he wants to make a break for it, he won't warn you like that," Jeff says. "The other day he tried to sneak out of bed. Didn't you, Dad?" He musters a sheepish smirk.

I summon his nurse Gloria, a broad-shouldered good old gal with a southern accent and a button dangling from her ID badge that says JESUS SAVES. She fiddles with his catheter and sings "It Is Well With My Soul" while Jeff and I discreetly look away, effectively deflating any remaining delusions I may have had that this was going to be some poignant movie scene. It turns out that except for my horribly unkempt hair and two inches of roots, dying is nothing like *Terms of Endearment.*

We sit together for the rest of the morning, all four of us, as Dad drifts in and out of seemingly multiple levels of awareness. He is sometimes very peaceful and often distressingly uncomfortable. Mom and Gloria have to make constant adjustments to his assorted tubes and drips. His voice is low and soft, but he keeps trying to talk.

He is agitated. "Agitated"—that's the word Gloria keeps using. "They usually become agitated right before they go. It's because he's traveling," she explains. "They go in and out between this world and the next." Do they? I don't know what they do. I don't know where they travel.

I watch Gloria as she goes through the routines of caretaking. She is competent and inspiringly brisk. But Dad is just another patient to her, another one of the departing, going through a checklist of expected actions before his final one. He's not the man who married her. He's not the man who raised her. He's not the man who loved her when her own father didn't. He's just another tourist in the airport lounge of death. A life of globe hopping, of pyramids climbed and rivers sailed, and now, Dad is taking one last trip. I hope the destination is blissful, because the journey is a bitch.

In a calmer moment, Dad turns in my direction, and his gaze seems remarkably bright and knowing. He looks at me like he's looking at me for the first time. Or like he knows he's looking at me for the last time. "Such pretty eyes," he says at last, and he pulls me in for a kiss. The plastic tubing running out of his nose bumps my cheek.

"You too," I say.

Around the time we would have eaten lunch if anybody were still eating lunch these days, an intern comes in and checks on him, then gently takes us aside. "His vitals are slipping," she says. "It's likely only 24 to 48 hours now."

There's no more putting off the inevitable anymore. Dad is going to die imminently, and that means I've got a BoltBus reservation to cancel.

I was supposed to visit Debbie in Philadelphia this weekend. Debbie and I arranged it several weeks ago, soon after she started chemo. Mike and the boys are going down to Florida for spring training, and we were to have a girly weekend of art museums and window-shopping and elaborately strung-together profanities. I had paid for my bus ticket and made reservations for dinner at Le Virtù, our college friend Cathy's Italian restaurant in South Philly.

When Dad got sick, I knew it was highly improbable I would be able to make the trip, but I had told myself it was possible. Just a few days ago, Jeff and I were making plans for how he'd come home to take care of the girls for the one night I would be away. Then we were in Denial. Now we have to get into Acceptance.

"I'm sorry," Jeff says. "I know you were looking forward to seeing Debbie."

"Don't be stupid," I say. "I'm just glad I came here in time to hang out with Dad."

I have to get home to get the girls from school, so I go over to Dad's bed one last time. He's sleeping now, his breathing shallow but steady. I flash back to a spring night two decades ago, nervously meeting my boyfriend's parents for dinner. "I'm Jerry," he'd boldly said, "but you can call me Dad if you like." I'd never called anybody Dad before.

"Goodbye, Dad," I whisper. "I love you."

I make it out of the hospice, back onto a Metro-North full of U2 song–slurring midday drunks clad in green, onto the subway filled with more of the same, over to school pickup, and all the way home—clutching a broken cable box the whole time—before I start to fall apart.

"Why don't you watch *The Princess Diaries*?" I suggest to the kids as I close the bedroom door, and I pull myself together long enough to call Deb to cancel our weekend. "How's the chemo been going?" I ask hesitantly.

What you don't want to say to someone who's undergoing cancer treatment is anything that sounds like you're pressuring her to get better. No "Not much longer, right?" No "I thought you'd be done by now."

"They're telling me I have to get my CA 125 number down," she says. Cancer antigen 125 is a type of protein that's used as a marker for the presence of ovarian cancer. A number of 35 or under in your blood work is considered normal, but in ovarian cancer, normal is relative. "A few weeks ago it was down to 120," she says, "so I thought, swell, we'll be wrapping this up in no time. Then the next week it was up to 150. They keep telling me not to get hung up on the number. When you're saying I have to keep doing chemo until I get my number down, I think maybe you're the ones hung up on it."

"So, speaking of cancer," I say, because I am that brilliant with a segue, "Jeff's dad is going to go at any minute so I can't leave town."

She doesn't hesitate, not even a second. "It's like he didn't even think about us," she says.

"I know," I reply. "He's such a ruiner. I promise I'll come down when he's dead."

"All right," she says, "but then you're going to have to put up with Mike and the boys."

"Just for that, I'm bringing Jeff and the girls," I say. "Two can play that game."

"I guess I'll see you soon, then," she says.

"See you soon," I answer, and then I put down the phone and sob like a child until Anne Hathaway assumes the title of heir to the throne of Genovia.

Friday comes, and though Dad is lapsing out of consciousness more frequently, he is still hanging on. The logistical challenge of another weekend of solo parenting is the least of it—the girls and I know how to function capably as a trio. We had plenty of experience the period Jeff and I were separated, and we've been crushing it all month. This time, however, the mood is sadder and more ominous. "Can't we visit Grandpa?" they ask, and it kills me to tell them it's not a good idea.

"He's very sick and very weak," I explain. "He can't speak, and he's really out of it with the medicine. You can make him cards."

So Lucy draws a diagram called "My Grandpa" mapped out with the words "Funny. Generous. Kind." Bea meanwhile scrawls "I love you" and draws a sunny picture of the two of them together. They're beautiful. He will never rouse enough to see them.

Our school's art teacher has a trip to the Museum of Modern Art planned for Saturday, so we immerse ourselves in an afternoon getaway of beauty. We stand, awed, in front of Van Gogh's "Starry Night." As the children sprawl in front of a Jackson Pollock, Bea raises her hand to share something with the group. "My grandfather is a wonderful artist," she says, "but his stuff isn't like this." I bask in the pride in her eyes, savoring the fact that for today, she can still talk about her grandfather in the present tense.

We go home, and I make pancakes and bacon for dinner, because, why not. Afterward, we stride on to the baseball field by our building, where our astronomer friend Jason has set up his telescope so we can look at the sky. Tonight the moon is the closest it has been to Earth in 18 years, and it's big and bright and at least for tonight beats the pants off anything in Times Square. But there are other wonders in the sky.

"Look over here," Jason says, as he spins the telescope in the direction toward a far-off nebula. I peer through the telescope and gasp in astonishment at the sight of distant miracles. Somewhere on the other side of the universe, stars are being born. This is where we all come from. This is where we all go.

The days go by, and still Dad does not die. He is not going gently. I'm beginning to doubt he's going at all. The thing nobody ever told me about having someone close to you die is that it can get downright boring.

"My father hung on for ten days after they said it was the end," says Shannon as she and I stand shivering in the schoolyard on a frigid afternoon as our children romp, stubbornly oblivious of the elements.

"Christ," I say. "It's like when I went two weeks past my due date with Bea."

"It takes a lot of work to come into this world," she says, "and it takes a lot of work to leave it."

On Wednesday night, the girls and I have a camping trip in the living room. I cook up hot dogs and we make s'mores in the microwave and we tell stories, and eventually we spread out to sleep together on a pile of pillows in the middle of the floor.

At 3 a.m., I bolt upright, wide awake, unfathomably unnerved. It's as if I'd heard a strange sound in the apartment, or forced myself awake from a nightmare, but I didn't. I get up and check on the children, peck them each on their sleeping cheeks, and stumble back to restless sleep.

In the morning, there is a light dusting of fresh snow on the ground. Apparently Mother Nature didn't get the memo that we're three days into spring now. I somnambulantly move through our routines. Breakfasts are consumed and dishes piled up. Teeth and hair are brushed. The girls and I walk together in near total silence to school, and I trudge back in the unseasonably bitter cold with my neighbor Ciaran, talking about the upcoming school spring break. It isn't until I'm back home and emptying my pockets that I notice the new voice mail on my phone. "It's me," the voice says. "Call me when you get the chance." Jeff doesn't need to say any more; the message is already there in the tone in his voice.

I tell my editor I'm taking a day off, and call Jeff to check in. He and his mother have already been busy with arrangements. He says it happened around 6:30 this morning and that it was peaceful. "We just left the funeral home," he says. "So now I'm going to grab a latte and hit the cemetery. I have to say that after watching what dying of cancer looks like, I'm seriously hoping for a heart attack."

"Oh, totally," I tell him. "I am all about getting hit by a bus. Which," I add, "is also my retirement plan."

Later, when I meet the girls at the school gate at dismissal time, I have a nervous smile frozen on my face. "Who wants cupcakes?" I ask, transparently. "How about some big chocolate chip cookies?" I take them over to Beans and Vines and sit them down. "Sky's the limit. Whatever you want." The girls look at each other nervously. They know this is Mommy's stupid way of telling them that Grandpa is dead. So they rightfully exploit my vulnerability and demand cupcakes the size of their heads. I reach across the table and put one hand on Lucy's hand and one on Bea's. "Grandpa passed away this morning," I say. They don't look surprised. They don't cry. They are as tired as I am.

The next day Jeff comes home, drained and in need of his best suit. And this time, when he goes back out to his parents' house, he's bringing all of us. We pack our bags and follow him in a somber procession toward the Metro-North train. We bring the pictures the girls drew for Grandpa, to put in his casket.

Mom ushers us into the house. It's the first time the girls and I have been there since we came out for the girls' birthday two months ago. Everything looks just the same, but everything feels entirely different. We hang up our coats in the hall closet, wedging them in among Dad's jackets. The sight of them hits me sharply. Death isn't just about loss. It's about absence. Loss happens once. Absence is the rest of your life. It's never hearing a voice on the phone again. It's an empty chair at the dinner table. It's coats that will never again be worn.

After Jeff and I get unpacked, I find Lucy standing in the kitchen crying, with Bea fused to her in a hug. Lucy is in a moral crisis. She wants to go to the wake and she doesn't want to go to the wake. "I don't know what to do," Lucy says. "I don't want to see Grandpa looking all different, but I want to say goodbye one last time. I want to be strong."

"You are strong," I say. "You are so strong. If seeing Grandpa will upset you, then don't do it. If it'll make you feel better, then go ahead. Just don't think you have to do anything for me or Daddy or anybody else. It's about what you need, okay?"

Bea chimes in philosophically. "You know Grandpa isn't really there, right, Lucy? Grandpa is gone. What's left—that's just his clothes."

She nods. "I do. I'm just not sure I can see it."

Bea, meanwhile, has decided she does not want to see what's left of Grandpa, and I am cool with my seven-year-old skipping the sight of her dead, cancer-ravaged grandfather. Tonight she and I will stay back at the house, receiving a steady stream of roast chickens and fruit baskets.

Later, as Jeff is straightening his tie, Lucy slips upstairs and dons her black velvet Christmas dress, the one with the taffeta ruffle and the wonky zipper.

"Are you sure?" I ask as I pull the zipper up slowly and hope that it doesn't, like this entire month, go completely off the rails.

"I'm sure," she says. "I want to be with Daddy."

By the time Jeff, Lucy, and Mom return in the evening, Bea is fast asleep and I am in my pajamas watching *The House Bunny* on TV. Though I had expected that Lucy would return thoroughly exhausted, I had not anticipated this fresh new air of drowsy loveliness about her. She looks older, and absolutely beautiful. She parks herself on the couch and rests her head on my shoulder. "Mommy," she says with a heavy sigh.

"How was it?" I ask.

"It was surreal," she replies. "Grandpa was there, but he looked really different." She pauses. "I met the mayor. I talked to people about how I'm playing Prospero in *The Tempest* at school."

She's grown up so much this year. Part of her childhood, the one that didn't yet know sickness and death, is gone. "You know," I say, "you're always so good and so kind. When a kid is kind, it's usually because she feels like being kind. Today, you were there for your family. You were kind because you were needed." She places her hand in mine. "Mommy," she sighs again, sleepily.

The next morning, the morning of the funeral, the family goes to the church and files into our pew at the front. Lucy wears her velvet dress again, because we don't exactly have a closetful of dressy mourning apparel. Bea is in her darkest dress as well. Undeterred by the fact that it's sleeveless, she resourcefully packed something to wear underneath. It's a roller derby jersey I bought her a few months ago. Under that prim navy blue frock, she's sporting a shirt emblazoned with the words MAYHEM FOREVER.

Bea swings her hair playfully as she plops down between Jeff and me, while Lucy somberly places herself on my right. There's maturity to Lucy already, but though I know Bea adored her grandfather, she so far seems blessedly less troubled by the loss. We sing hymns and say prayers. Jeff gets up and nervously begins the eulogy.

"I was so worried about what to say," he says, "then I remembered, a half hour after this is over, nobody will remember anything I said anyway." But I will. I'll remember how he credits his father with teaching him to be a father himself. How he praised his generosity. How he stressed that the support his father gave so freely wasn't an accident; it was a conscious act. "Love," he says, "is a choice."

Jeff and I learned that the hard way when our marriage fell apart, when we realized that love is either something you actively do every day or it isn't. We learned it a new way when we reconciled. I can pinpoint the moment I knew we had a real chance of making it work a second time. It was when we'd gone on a big date late last spring. He had told me then, "I used to think the relationship part of my life was settled and I never had to worry about it. Now I think, if you love someone, you have to take it one day at a time. And you have to work at it one day at a time." Love is an ever renewing contract. It's a choice you make—and keep making. You make it when you learn to change a woman's bandages. You make it when you show up to watch your father die.

Then Dad's friend Will, his former church organist, gets up to say a few words of introduction before sitting down at the piano. "This was one of Jerry's favorites," he explains. As he launches into Brahms's op. 118, Intermezzo no. 2 in A major, the room erupts in sobs. The music is so sublime; it cannot fail to move the assembly. As tears are streaming down my face, I notice Lucy out of the corner of my eye, wiping her cheeks. I put my arm around her and she buries herself into my chest, shuddering as I stroke her hair. Then, ever stoic, she takes a deep, composing breath before she picks herself up and turns back to face the front.

I look next over to Bea, and she turns her little face up to me. Her eyes are shining with tears, but she's smiling. It's a dazzling vision, seeing her enraptured with the tenderness of the moment. This is my Bea—the girl who can quite literally smile through the tears. This, too, is grief—pain and release and the most peculiar, astonishing sweetness. It's like a journey to the bottom of the ocean. It's dark in this place that the rest of the world seldom sees. But it's full of extraordinary, luminous beauty too. It is, in its own way, a marvel.

CHAPTER 10

Spring Breakthrough

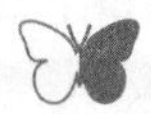

April 2011

I always play a game when I'm waiting for the elevator. It's called, "Patient, Caregiver, or Staff?"

Sometimes it's easy. The very old, the ones clutching a child's hand, the ones in concealing scarves and hats and obvious wigs, the ones so fragile they have to sit resignedly on the bench in the elevator for just the short duration of the ride—they're eliminated right away. Likewise the ones in white coats and hospital ID badges. Then it gets harder. What to make of the gray-haired African-American man in the blazer and tie? Or the stylish 30-something brunette with the Prada handbag? Or the thin, bald Middle Eastern man staring resolutely at the floor? I watch my fellow passengers sizing me up too, observing the way I nod casually to the security guard and unhesitatingly hit the elevator button without consulting the directory. I don't look like one of the sick, unless you can see the patch of bare flesh on my head. I note whether our eyes meet in wordless fraternity. We always try to find each other, don't we? Because you're one of us or you're one of them.

I step into the waiting room, and when I take off my coat, my MSKCC uniform—black jeans and my FUCK CANCER shirt—makes clear which side I'm on. I sit, observing another one of us now. She's a skeletal woman in a wheelchair, being pushed slowly toward the restroom. She looks no more than 20. She also looks about 80. There's another. An old man muttering to no one in particular, "It smells like sickness in here. Mine, mostly." There's a Rivers Cuomo type in nerd glasses with a clipped, geeky rhythm to the way he speaks to the woman accompanying him. His wife, I guess. If it weren't for the uneven patchy tufts all over his head, he'd look like any Williamsburg artist. Maybe even with them. "Not all babies are cute," I hear him saying, "but ours definitely is." Now he's talking about dinner tomorrow, and trying to figure out what he will and won't be able to eat. Across from me, there's a young lady in a bright red pageboy wig.

It's my first time back to Sloan Kettering since Dad's death three weeks ago. Outside, midtown is a riot of April beauty—every spindly tree in front of every enormous building is pimped out in a flurry of white blossoms. Inside, I am crunching on a compost cookie from Milk Bar and feeling lots of cancer feelings while I watch Red Pageboy munch a cupcake. By any means necessary, I think.

I'm back for another checkup, part of my routine maintenance now. I don't care how pleasant the facility is; I dread going, every time. I hate wearing the gown. It infantilizes me; it makes me a patient instead of just a person. This morning I'd reluctantly told Jeff, "I have to accept the idea that this is a long-term situation for me now."

He'd said, "Beats the hell out of a short-term one." That's the hope, anyway. I like to think the odds of that being true are getting better.

Earlier this month, the National Cancer Institute announced that 27 sites across the country, including Sloan Kettering, would participate in its newly formed Cancer Immunotherapy Trials Network—a multicenter research group dedicated to exploring immune system–based cancer treatments and "to select, design, and conduct early-phase trials." Prophetically for future drug combination patients like me, principal investigator Martin A. "Mac" Cheever noted at the time, "One of the difficulties in developing cancer immunotherapy agents is that the drugs are not likely to do much on their own, but will need to be used in combinations of two or more. The reason for this is that T cells, the immune cells that have the potential to specifically attack cancer cells, need to be selectively activated, expanded in number, and stimulated to survive long-term. It is unlikely that a single compound could accomplish all of these steps, especially as the treatments will also need to override the natural checks and balances our bodies have in place to prevent overexpansion of T cells."

Not that single compounds are out of the game—far from it. On March 25—exactly one day after Dad died—a story in the *New York Times* had caught my eye. It was about how "The first drug shown to prolong the lives of people with the skin cancer melanoma" had won approval from the Food and Drug Administration that day. The treatment, ipilimumab—also known by its Bristol-Myers Squibb brand name Yervoy—is the first new melanoma drug approved by the FDA in more than a decade. It works differently from conventional cancer treatment, by activating the patient's immune system to destroy deadly disease cells. It's the drug Dr. Esposito told me about last fall.

Cancer cells set off inhibitory mechanisms in our invader-fighting T cells. But a protein receptor called CTLA-4, which lives on the surface of those T cells, can be manipulated. That's what ipilimumab does. It's what's known as a monoclonal antibody therapy (that's what the "mab" in ipilimumab stands for), using antibodies made—and copied—in a lab, and then introduced into the patient to release the CTLA-4 braking system—so the T cells can attack the cancer.

Ipilimumab is also unusual—and controversial—for its astronomically high cost and its still relatively low survival rate. The current protocol is four treatments, and the price tag is—holy crap—around $120,000, a price tag that Dr. James Allison himself will later refer to in a newspaper interview as "obscene." I assume it's made of pixie blood and treasures from the lost city of Atlantis.

For that kind of money, for what Bristol-Myers Squibb notes in its press release is "the first and only drug therapy for melanoma to demonstrate significant improvement in survival," you think you'd be getting a sure thing. Then you'd read the part boasting: "Median survival was ten months." When you're dealing with a deadly disease, just getting a little extra time is enough to be considered a triumph. But the kicker—the thing harder to discern in the midst of the media blitz—is that intriguingly, there are people on Yervoy who get much more.

The *New York Times* story notes, "More than 20 percent of the people who received Yervoy in the trial lived at least two years." That's not the kind of statistic that inspires loads of confidence. But this is the part that's interesting. Trials have to have end points. The data won't necessarily tell you about the people who live much, much longer. And the appeal of immunotherapy is that when it works, it looks like it really works. It's like what William Coley saw more than a century ago—a population of patients who get better and stay better. That includes patients who get better without technically being cured.

The approval of Yervoy represents a small yet seismic shift in the way cancer is being viewed and treated. It's a newer perspective, with an emphasis on overall survival. And it's a treatment that doesn't involve the typical grueling, traumatizing rigors of hair loss and nausea—protocols so rigorous and daunting that, as one of my oncology nurses says, patients are often scared off treatment entirely. "They see people who've lost their hair and lost weight, people who are throwing up. They don't want to look sick." That's one of the many funny things about cancer—it's often the treatment, not the disease itself, that makes you feel like hell. Heck, I walked around all last summer feeling just fine, while my melanoma was quietly burrowing its way into my head.

"Mary Williams?" says an administrator who looks exactly like George Michael, circa the Thatcher years. I cannot even be bothered to correct him.

Soon, I am sitting on the edge of the exam table in my seersucker as an intern I've never met before pads his fingertips around my neck, checking my lymph nodes. "Now go like this," he says, putting his elbows straight out to the side and his hands up in the air, like he's modeling for a hieroglyph. I take a deep nervous breath, and he begins to probe around the nodes under my arms. I instinctively swat him away, and then dissolve into helpless, shrieking giggles.

"Okay, so you're ticklish," he says.

"I apologize," I reply. "I can do this." I put up my arms again. As soon as he moves toward me, I clamp them shut again, and I'm laughing so hard now I can barely breathe. "This never happens," I explain sheepishly. "I'm going to think very sad thoughts now. I just had a death in my family, so that should help." I raise my arms up again and bite my lip, contemplating how much my children's education IRA has depreciated recently and how rapidly the rain forest is disappearing. "Your hands could be warmer," I say, squirming like mad while tittering uncontrollably as he proceeds to prod around my groin. I try to make light, distracting conversation. "Is melanoma going to be your specialty?"

"Actually," he says, "I'm pursuing colon cancer."

"Well, you won't get a lot of laughs when you do those exams," I say. He looks considerably less amused than I am as he scrawls on a clipboard and exits hastily.

Dr. Partridge comes in to go over my last labs and scans and to do some follow-up poking around. "Everything looks great," she says. "You still have these two growths on your lung. They're very small, but we need to keep an eye on them. We'll check again in July. They could be scar tissue, or benign growths." Or, though she doesn't come out and say it, cancer.

Although much depends on factors including a person's initial staging and treatment, melanoma has a comeback rate that could rival Robert Downey, Jr.'s. Doctors often speak of recurrence in terms not of if but when. People who've already had melanoma are nine times likelier to develop new melanomas than those who have not. The Cleveland Clinic Center for Continuing Education estimates that "Despite adequate surgical resection of the primary melanoma, approximately 15 percent to 36 percent of patients with Stages 1 and 2 melanoma will have some form of recurrence or metastasis during their clinical course." In other words, the expectation that I will have cancer again is ever present.

After my appointment, I go down the street to a vegetarian restaurant for a steamy bowl of pea soup and a roll, and to bury my nose in Nathaniel Philbrick's *Mayflower*. I learned early on in this cancer adventure to make a special day of it when I go to Sloan Kettering. It takes a daunting amount of emotional energy, and afterward all I'm usually good for is weeping and ice cream. Debbie likewise has a routine—for her, it's all about those South Philly Italian sandwiches near her treatment facility.

Ever since our thwarted weekend in March, Deb and I have been trying to figure out a time to reschedule, something that won't conflict with her sons' Little League practice or a close family member dying. As I do a quick email check before heading home, I see she's sent me not only some dates in May but also some exceptionally good news. "The doctor says I have only two more chemo treatments to go. Then it's a year of the drugs. She even says my hair should come back pretty quickly." I'm sure a year of medication is no picnic, but it says that there's another year to be had. It says that there will be a 2012. "Jeff and the kids are welcome too," she adds. "Mike and the boys would like to see them." It's not the one-on-one chick weekend I'd originally envisioned, but it might be very therapeutic for Mike and Jeff to spend some time together.

CHAPTER 11

Wig Out

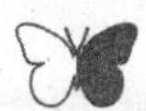

May 2011

It feels like the season turned to summer overnight. There's something about the change, and moving on, that's both wonderful and terrible. It snowed the morning Dad died. Now, as the temperatures rise, the grief is subsiding, but there's a strange guilt too. There's comfort in staying in place. It makes you feel close to the one who's gone. Moving on can feel like forgetting, and bring surprising new jabs of pain. I'm getting used to the bittersweet, though. Like seeing Deb and her family this weekend.

As the end of her chemo had approached, I'd sent Debbie a congratulatory gift—a print emblazoned with the words BAD HAIR DAY. Then, just two weeks ago, she'd called. "They found a two-centimeter tumor on my vaginal cuff," she told me. She's starting a new round of chemo soon, this time with Avastin. I have decided she's going to be okay, because she has to be okay.

As we pull into Debbie's drive, I spy a lanky, bespectacled, dark-haired figure through the window. For a crazy split second, I think it's her. Of course it's not. It's her son Tim. The bald lady coming out the front door, the one with no eyebrows and the Steven Van Zandt scarf action, that's Debbie.

"Welcome to our shit show," she says as she ambles toward the car, and my children tumble out of it. The last time we got together was 14 months ago. I'd come down to Philly in the midst of what turned out to be a ludicrous nor'easter that destroyed my umbrella and soaked through my luggage. We'd practically blown all the way to our friend Cathy's restaurant, shivering and famished, but when the food arrived, Debbie complained of a stomachache and could barely touch anything. For Halloween, she'd dressed as Medusa, just days before the diagnosis. I've got to give her credit—she's damn near cinematic in her ominous portents.

We regard each other almost sheepishly now. We've seen each other drunk and walk of shamed and pregnant, but with cancer? This is new. "Hey now," I tell her, as we part from an awkward hug, "your arms are so smooth."

"You should see my legs," she replies.

"I'm sure your entire bathing suit area is like a porn star's," I retort.

Mike, meanwhile, slaps Jeff on the back. "Hey man, I'm sorry. When all this happened, I really kept meaning to reach out to you," he says. "I would have if I wasn't so lazy."

"Yeah, me too," he replies.

Deb and I feed the kids first, dishing out grilled cheese sandwiches hot off the panini press while Jeff and Mike bond. Then, after the children have eaten, the grown-ups sit together outside at the big picnic bench, munching on crackers and the Rice Krispie treats I've brought.

"I lost my job," Mike says. "Same day they found Deb's new tumor." Then he breaks into a sardonic chuckle as Jeff's and my jaws drop. "Yeah," he says. "I was saving that one for when you got here."

"Can you believe it?" Debbie says. "Hey, let's lay off the guy whose wife has cancer."

"People have been very generous, though" says Mike. "When someone gets sick or you lose your job, you get all these lasagnas." He thinks a moment. "I hate lasagna now."

"We got potpies," I tell him. "First it was the cancer potpies and then it was the dead dad potpies. They got us through some rough days, and I never want to look at another potpie again."

In the afternoon, the kids run around Mike and Deb's big house and their big yard. They clamber up into the tree house; they go bananas on the trampoline. At a certain point I find myself jumping along with them. Debbie's son Adam does effortless somersaults, but the girls and I stick to chasing each other around, leaping ever higher and higher. I feel weightless and free.

"It's all been hard on Mike," Debbie says later. "He's so frustrated."

"When it's your own cancer, it's tough because you feel like you have no control over what's happening to you," I tell her. "Seeing it with you and with Dad, I get it now that when it's someone you love, it's a different kind of tough. Because then you really have no control."

Later we go to the local Strawberry Festival, where there are sack races and pie-baking contests and a fire truck just for climbing around on. Lucy correctly guesses the number of candies in a giant jar and wins them, a triumph for the visiting team.

As the fair winds down, Deb and I take off to have dinner together at Cathy's restaurant. "Don't get cancer," we yell in unison to Mike and Jeff. "Unless you already have it!" We guffaw as the car roars away.

On the drive, we talk, just a couple of cancer club ladies alone. It's then that Debbie tells me at last the full story of her diagnosis, and all about her former doctor.

"I hate that woman," she says. "I was having problems for months—months. Remember?" I do. "I got deathly sick in February of last year. That was the beginning of the symptoms. My doctor didn't even want to look at me. She told me to stop drinking milk. She said, 'When you get to be our age, a lot of women become lactose intolerant.'"

"Turns out you were cancer intolerant," I say.

"Then I went in for tests in the spring and she said, 'We found some cysts. Let's wait and see.' She told me to take Tums. Finally, at the end of the summer, I went in for a regular appointment and I said I was still having problems. She said they'd remove the cysts laparoscopically. I'll never forget it. She said, 'If that's what you want.'" You bet, that's what she wanted. I hate to imagine what would have happened if she hadn't.

"It was during the surgery they found the cancer," she continues, "and my doctor decided to try to take it out right there instead of closing me up and sending me to a real cancer doctor. She had no business whatsoever doing what she did. It was like the Keystone Cops operating on me. When I woke up, it was, 'Oh, I'm so sorry, you have cancer in your ovaries and you also have it in your abdomen and I saw something on your liver.' "

"That. Bitch." I say.

"Then the nurse said, 'I'll pray for you,' and I thought, I don't want you to pray for me, I want you to treat me. Later, when I got hooked up with my gyn-onc and went to the hospital for the full hysterectomy, you know, doctors are always trying to cover their asses, but he read some stuff off the chart out loud." She hesitates, like she's not sure she wants to continue. "This is so disgusting. I can't even think about it," she says. "One of the ovaries came out fine. The other was 'compromised.' That's what it said. When she took it out, something happened, and now there are all these cancer cells swimming around in my blood. My new doctor said the cancer was probably not self-contained and already in my blood anyway, but I just picture this cancerous ovary, dripping back into my body."

I picture it too, and I don't know whether to be enraged or just really, really sad.

"I hope there's a hell," I say, "so that dismissive butcher of yours can go there."

The next morning, I wander into Debbie's bedroom looking for towels. Debbie is in her bathroom, inspecting her cranium. "Look at this," she says. She has a few stubby gray hairs that have come in on her head since the last chemo ended. Before the next one starts. "Goddammit, now I'm gray. What if it all comes in like this when this is all over?" Debbie is not a touchy-feely person, but I cannot stop myself from reaching out and rubbing her nearly bare head. It's a little prickly and pleasant, like when you let your legs go for a while. It's the aftermath of a calamity, and the fresh canvas for a new one.

"That reminds me—want to meet Ellen?" she asks, and she leads me out of the bathroom toward the bookcase in her bedroom. There, on the top shelf, is a plain mannequin head with a brunette wig that looks like the doll hair version of Debbie's old haircut.

"There she is," she says. "I hate this bitch too."

"Hi," I say. "I've heard a lot about you, Ellen. I thought you'd be taller." I turn to Deb. "Why did you name her Ellen?"

"It's her name," she says. "It was on the box. I got her at the Cancer Lady store."

"You have a Cancer Lady store in town?" I say.

"Yeah," she says. "I drive past it every day. It's called Lovely You."

"That," I say, "is the most terrible thing I've ever heard."

We need to get back home, and Deb and her family have their own Sunday engagements, so we pack up our toothbrushes and take a few last photographs. On the way out of town, we all go to the ball field to drop off the boys at Little League, and to say hello to Debbie's parents too. I've known them as long as I've known Debbie. I still think of us as the kids and them as the grown-ups, even though I'm now the age they were when Deb and I first met. Deb's mom, Clara, always still talks to me like I'm the teenager she feels she should take care of, the girl sleeping over at her house. I love her for that. We say our goodbyes while the boys play ball, and I'm totally fine until Clara hugs me—a big, fierce hug that I know is as much for Deb as it is for me. When she releases me from it, her eyes are red and moist.

"Well, that was fun and profoundly heavy," says Jeff as I sit in the passenger side, looking on my camera at the photos from the weekend. There's one that gets me. A picture from this morning of four smiling, silly children on a bright green lawn. Four children who a year ago had never considered the possibility of losing their mothers. Four children whose lives have been rewritten.

"Now you cheer up and dry your tears," Jeff tells me. "Then next weekend we can celebrate my dead father's birthday."

June 2011

"How are you doing?" my dermatologist asks cautiously. It's now my first summer after my ill-fated best summer ever. "I've been keeping in touch with your doctors at Sloan Kettering. Let me make sure I have all your information right. You just had surgery, no chemo, right?"

"So far, so good," I say.

"That's amazing," Dr. Silver replies. "Because that was a very serious melanoma."

I know the truth—that escaping chemo means almost nothing when it comes to melanoma. It doesn't mean I was amazing. It means

I was without other options. I look down at my crappy, crinkly pink ensemble. "The gowns are much nicer at Sloan Kettering," I tell her. Then I add, "I've watched two people I love go through some serious cancer this year, and I'm really glad you're my doctor."

"Thanks," she says. "You're very lucky."

"That's what people keep telling me," I reply.

I suppose I am. What if I'd put off going to the doctor last summer? What if I had gone and Dr. Silver wasn't as on the ball as she was? What if she'd been like Debbie's doctor and blown me off? What if I didn't have insurance? Incredibly, in all of this, I did luck out. I don't assume, however, that means my luck is infinite. I usually try not to let myself have such thoughts, but it's hard not to when you're wearing a dumb paper dress.

I'm glad Dr. Silver can acknowledge that my cancer was serious, even as she's reminding me how fortunate I am. Lately, it's been downright odd how spectacularly some people I know have been failing at cancer conversation. A common refrain is "How are you doing? You're all cured now? Right, anyway . . ." and then a change of subject. I haven't known what to say in response. I'm not even a year into this. I usually just reply, "I hope I'm well." Because it's not my job to make anybody else feel comfortable about my trip to Cancer Town.

Dr. Silver runs her hands along my flesh. "Have you always had this mole?" she asks, pointing to a freckle on my hand.

"Yes," I say, taking a wild guess. I'm Irish. I have a galaxy of freckles on my shoulders alone. I couldn't possibly catalog all of them. Today I just care about one. "Take a look at this," I tell her, pointing to a small scab on my collarbone.

"It looks benign," she tells me, "but we'll biopsy it. I want to biopsy that thing on your forehead too." What thing on my forehead?

A day later, Dr. Silver calls back. I know not to flip out because this time she doesn't tell me she's sorry. "It is skin cancer, but it's not serious," she says. Ten months ago, this was my worst scenario version of the conversation we'd have. It is laughable.

"It's a superficial basal cell carcinoma. We have two options: We can do a scrape and burn, which is less invasive, or we can surgically cut it out." Funnily enough, "scrape and burn" doesn't sound non-invasive to my hearing. "It's completely unrelated to the melanoma on your head. Just know that you can have more carcinoma and melanomas locally. Don't get too concerned, hardly anybody ever dies of this." Then she catches herself. "I hope you don't mind that I put it that way."

"Oh, please," I tell her. "After what I've been through, this will be a piece of cake."

A week later I don my peacock print dress, robin's egg blue high heels, a big hat adorned with a hot pink silk flower, and enormous sunglasses for my procedure. Before I leave in the morning, Bea busts out her toy magic wand. "You will be fine," she says, waving it authoritatively toward my throat. "You are fiiine." It's not quite a Patronus Charm, but it'll do.

"How are the girls?" Dr. Silver asks as she plunges a long needle deep into the place right above my heart. I feel an iciness that, impossibly, seems to shoot right down to my toes as I grit my teeth and look at the ceiling. Her assistant hands her a tool that looks like a coke spoon. As she scrapes off the flesh, I can hear the *scritch scritch scritch* of instrument on skin, feel the tug of it whittling off layers. Then, *zap,* begins the burning part. That's me I smell now, frying up with a wisp of smoke and the unmistakable stinging stink of burnt flesh. "It'll dissipate in a few seconds," she says. "Just hold your breath."

"I've been holding my breath for a year now," I say. Finally, she pulls the tool away. It's bright red now, and there's a lumpy pink-and-white mass of my poisoned skin on it. She taps it into a vial. "See?" she says. "There it is."

"That's disgusting," I reply. I'm a repulsive, seeping, shedding thing, like Jeff Goldblum in *The Fly*.

"All done," she answers with motherly tenderness as she applies a bandage. "You want the Scarguard?" she asks, and I'm down another $65 for a small bottle of liquid and the small hope of someday having my collarbone look normal.

I get up, surprisingly woozy for having just had a routine office procedure. When I step out onto Broadway, the noise and the unseasonably scorching June heat assault me, and I'm feeling like tectonic plates are shifting beneath my feet. I totter to a nearby deli for a freshly squeezed orange juice, and the white-haired Italian counter guy regards my big hat and big sunglasses and drawls, "You look like a movie star. A mooooovie staaaar." I feel like a few miles of unpaved road.

The newly expanded second section of the High Line has just opened up, so I stroll slowly over and walk along it, sipping my juice and people-watching. In the ladies' room, an encouraging loop of positive affirmations plays as part of an auditory art installation. "You are in total harmony with the universe," I hear just before I flush. "Everything is fine," the bathroom tells me, and as I look in the mirror at my freshly bandaged, semibald body, I cannot suppress a laugh. If you say so, toilet. Everything is fiiiiine.

"It was no big deal," I tell Jeff when I call him from a bench overlooking Chelsea afterward. "I just got a Band-Aid." But that night, there's a dark look on his face as he hugs me when he comes through the door. "I'm so glad it was just benign. I couldn't have handled anything happening to you in the same year we lost Dad," he says.

I don't tell him what I'm thinking. That the year is only halfway over.

CHAPTER 12

Here It Comes Again

July 2011

"Are we going to see Grandpa's bones?" Bea asks excitedly.

"Not quite," Jeff replies.

We have detoured to the Stop & Shop en route to the cemetery, and the girls are busy bickering over their choices of spindly supermarket bouquets of carnations and roses. "These," I say, pointing to a bunch of gerbera daises. "He liked these."

We're spending the weekend at Jeff's mother's house. It's still odd not to think of it as his parents' house. It's odd that visiting the in-laws now means stopping by the cemetery, but that's where we're headed this morning. The family needs a lot of time together lately—Jeff and Mom especially—and Mom wants us to visit the grave.

It is a beautiful day to stop by where Dad is spending eternity. Dad's headstone still isn't there yet, just a small placard and a last name on the side of a twisting path. There is, however, to Mom's great vexation, a dried-up mixed bouquet encroaching on his space.

"That woman next to us," Mom says. "She has no sense of boundaries."

We stand together, solemnly gazing at the dirt. "Are we on top of Grandpa right now?" Bea asks.

"I suppose so," Jeff says.

Mom looks at the marker, her face touchingly serene. She's once again in the company of the man she loved. "When the doctor showed me his scans last summer," she says, "I could see that the cancer had gone all over. The doctor and I had a private conversation and he said, 'I'm afraid I don't have good news. I don't know how long it'll take, but it's terminal.' We still thought that he'd be stable for longer. We didn't think it would be so fast. We kept making plans. We talked about having a big party for his 80th birthday. Even near the end, when he'd say, 'Do you think I'm sick because of the cancer or the chemo?' I always tried to be encouraging."

"It's the only way to live," I say. "As long as you're breathing, what else is there to do but keep going?"

"I'll tell you this much," Mom says. "Tonight, I'm going to watch as many episodes of *The Golden Girls* as it takes."

I take photos of Jeff and Mom, their arms around each other and surrounded by headstones, smiling in the summer sun. Jeff and the girls lovingly place their flowers on top of the dirt. "We love you," Jeff says, his eyes moist with sorrow. Two days from now I will be looking at those dewy-eyed photos on my phone when Jeff will text me: "Turns out about Dad's grave: Not where they told us it was." I guess it's the thought that counts.

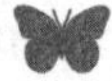

In the afternoon, we take the girls down to the lake, where they splash around until their lips turn blue and their skin is pruney, their sunscreen melting off in the water. "Dad would have loved all of this," Jeff says. "I know he had a good life. I know he had a full life. He just wanted more."

"This mortality stuff is nuts," I say. "You live in the world, you love people, and then they die. You love the world. Then you die. What's up with that?"

"Let's go get an ice cream," Jeff says, walking in the direction of the Good Humor truck. "I see a Choco Taco that is totally going to make me forget all about my dead dad." And we hold hands as we amble in the direction of the brief oblivion of frozen dairy.

Later, Mom and I set out to go errand running, giving me the suburban thrill of shopping for economy-size jugs of Tide in a car with a roomy trunk. As we head out to drive to the store, Mom looks at Dad's photo on the sideboard. "We're going out to dinner at Abatino's tonight and we're going to have a good time," she tells it. "I wish you could be here with us. But if you were, you wouldn't be able to come anyway, would you? Damn cancer." I think this is the first time I've ever heard her say the word "damn."

In the car, Mom and I talk about the changes in both our lives since cancer stomped in. "So many people have been wonderful," she says, "and I want to accept help when I need it." Fortunately, the woman who was voted most popular in her high school graduating class is really good at reaching out. "I've had family in Kentucky invite me to visit, neighbors ask if I want to go out to dinner. That's been good for me," she says. The response has been uneven, though. One of her closest friends hasn't been in touch since the funeral "Robin?" she says, "Nothing. It's surprising."

Disasters don't just show you what you're made of. They show you, with savage clarity, what everybody else is made of too. I learned this for the first time when Jeff and I separated and I no longer fit in among the local Perfect Mom set. I learned it again this year. Not everyone will be there when you're so broken you're not sure who you are anymore. The worst part is that they will provide, when you need it least, fresh grief to contend with. They're the losses within a loss. Olivia was the hardest.

I met Olivia several years and many hairstyles ago. We traveled together and cried at movies next to each other and endured breakups and always came running when the other had a crisis. Our bond was profound. She was one of the first people I told when I got cancer. She sent a floral arrangement and that, aside from a few superficial emails, has been that. I get that it's awkward and scary for everybody. When life drags you through illness or trauma, it's an adjustment for the people around you too. They have to get used to this new person walking around in your old skin—or what's left of it. And it will turn out that not everybody wants to get to know that person or relates well to her. That post-cancer, post-widowhood, postwar version of yourself may just not be everybody's cup of tea. Then again, the post-divorce, post–job loss version of them may not be not your cup of tea either. You lose people along the way. But it hurts nonetheless.

"Maybe Robin assumed that if I needed something, I'd ask," Mom says.

"Needing to ask isn't the point, is it?" I reply, and she nods. It reminds me of my friend Evan, whose boyfriend admiringly told her after she'd had major surgery that she was so good at taking care of herself—and how she knew right then that they were finished. Just because you can take care of yourself doesn't mean you always ought to. The friends who've moved my heart most deeply in all of this have been the ones who didn't wait for a request. I'm still trying to forgive the ones who let me down. "I've learned," I continue, "that some of the people I trusted most in the world just aren't good in a crisis. But from here on in, I'm sticking like glue to the ones who are."

It's not yet 8 a.m., and it's already a sweltering, sticky New York City morning. I am briskly hoofing it across midtown, trying to make it in time for another spin of routine CT scans and tests around Sloan Kettering.

The receptionist on the eighth floor beams brightly when she sees me. "Good morning, Ms. Williams," she says. I like her. I know her. It also depresses me that I'm a regular to her now.

She sends me over to the gentleman on the other side of the desk. "Hello, my name is Sal," he drones in a monotone. "You're here today for a CT scan of your chest-abdomen-pelvis. Do you want your drink chilled or room temperature?"

"Rocks, salt, Patron," I reply.

"I'll put you down for room temperature," he continues flatly, handing me a jug of what looks and tastes like brightly colored sports drink. This is the beverage that has ruined my distance running experience—I can no longer drink Gatorade without experiencing just a touch of stomach turning, visceral, post-traumatic stress. I know what Sal's going to explain next, verbatim. "You need to drink down to the line," he says, and I mouth the words along, like I do when I'm getting the safety demonstration on an airplane. "In about 30 minutes someone will bring you back for your exam. If you have to use the ladies' room, it's to your right by the water fountain. Don't hold it in; it's not part of your exam," he mumbles on. "Do you understand?"

"You bet," I say, grabbing the bottle and preparing to chug. "I've won contests."

I settle in and flip through a magazine in the waiting room. There's an ad for pomegranate juice with the seductive come-on "Change your expiration date." Bitch, please.

I drink the nasty stuff, change into a gown, strap in to the IV, and hop on the table. It's all nauseating but relatively painless. It's also already crushingly routine.

It's also the least nerve-racking thing I'll do all week, as I plan to spend much of the next few days without any clothes on. Because I must be emitting a bucket list crossing-off kind of vibe these days, a painter friend and photographer friend, independently of each other, have both invited me to pose for them for new art projects they've been working on. Naked. I lost all my modesty halfway through the birth of Lucy and kept it off through the breast-feeding of two children, so all my subsequent exposure has simply been a matter of opportunity. I am neither young nor beautiful, but the advantage of that is not caring about being young and beautiful.

So I spend three afternoons standing on my friend Dylan's coffee table, wearing only a symbolic wide-brimmed hat and discussing apocalyptic scenarios and how we think we'd fare if New York City overnight became a Cormac McCarthy novel. The hardest part isn't the exposure; it's how surprisingly tiring standing still can be. Then I do it all over again at my friend Chris's photography studio. On a gray summer morning, I take the train to Nyack, where I have a day clad in only a pair of high heels. I've endured the better part of the past year undressing for strangers, but this one isn't brandishing an IV lock or an icy stethoscope. It's all mostly silly and spirited, a creative collaboration and a blessed reprieve from my usual rigors of disrobing for medical inspection. When you've been through an intense medical crisis, it's nice to have friends around to remind you that being naked can be fun. There's only one shot I find hard to pose for.

As Chris changes filters, I blot my lipstick. "Do you want to show me your head?" he asks.

I don't. It's the ugliest part of my body. It's my damaged goods. And that tells me it's important.

"Sure," I reply.

I am not only not wearing any clothing, I am about to do the unthinkably unflattering act of bending forward from the hips, thereby revealing my utter and obvious lack of abdominal muscle tone. But I don't care about that part. Behold a stomach that's been stretched to the limit by two large babies who both went past their due dates. Whatever. What's making me want to run out of the room and cry is my head. I take a low bow and pull the hair around the scabby scar away. I hear the click of a shutter. I have never felt more vulnerable. "Got it," Chris says.

I love and trust Chris so I know it's all okay. He's not thinking, "Oh, uggo." Yet damned if the hardest thing in the world isn't just to let yourself be seen, in all your devastation. I carry that scar with me every day now, and I no longer make a huge effort to conceal it. But it makes me feel like a freak, and that never goes away. I am daily reminded that it's hard for people to look at my head. It's hard for me to look at it, too. This is who I am now. This is what I've endured. This is what did not kill me. There is violent exquisiteness there. I just hope someday I can be proud of it.

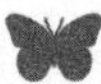

A few days after my scans and subsequent festival of nudity, I get a call. It's Carrie, the radiologist. "I'm looking at your scans," she says evenly, "and your latest results were troubling."

"Troubling," I think. That's better than "malignant," but nowhere near the ballpark of "fine."

"Those spots we found on your lung back in October have grown," she continues. "The lower lobe nodule has grown from four millimeters to six, and the upper one has grown from two millimeters to seven. They're still very small, and it could mean any number of things. But because they're getting bigger, what concerns me is that it could mean some melanoma broke away and traveled into your lung."

My stomach rapidly hurtles toward my feet. Ohfuckohfuckohfuckohfuckmylife. I am not a hypochondriacal Googler of bad news. I have tried hard to avoid horror stories about melanoma, and to hope that my cancer is in the past tense. I have also been writing and speaking about the disease, so I know a few things. Because I need to. I know, for instance, what happens when melanoma goes into your organs. It's called metastasis, and you won't find a lot of happy scenarios related to it, even if the tumors are small. Medline.com will tell you that "Nearly any cancer can spread to the lungs . . . A cure is unlikely in most cases. It is rare for someone with metastatic cancer to the lungs to live more than five years." The American Cancer Society says that the five-year survival rate for someone with Stage 4 melanoma is about 15 percent, but notes cheerfully that the prognosis for melanoma is better if the cancer has spread only to other sites on the skin or lymph nodes and not to other organs. A 2011 report in the *Annals of Oncology,* using Sloan Kettering's own patient database, dryly notes that "Outcomes for patients with metastatic malignant melanoma are generally poor; median survival ranges from six to fifteen months." I cannot escape the implications here. In medical terms, if what's happening to me is indeed a recurrence, my long-term prognosis sucks out loud.

Yet Carrie is remarkably calm about it all. "Right now they're both still shy of a centimeter," she says, "so in nine months, the growth has been very slow. That's encouraging. Because of their size and location, I don't think a surgical biopsy would even be possible just yet." *Yet.* Surely one of the most portentous words in cancer. "You could just enjoy the rest of your summer and wait until your next scheduled scans in six months and see where you are then," she continues, "but because of your cancer's high recurrence rate, you might prefer to have a consult with Dr. Partridge." Tiny specks in my lung. Could be nothing, but they're growing. I'd say the idea of enjoying the rest of the summer is not an option anymore.

"Thanks for the information," I say. "Can you transfer me over to Dr. Partridge's office?"

I knew all along there would be good checkups and not-so-good checkups. Yet the achiever in me cannot help feeling like I've let down the team.

That night at dinner, I give Jeff and the kids the light version of the story—that my condition has changed a little, and that I'm going back to meet with Dr. Partridge. It's easier to spring on them than "I could have cancer in my lungs, you guys."

"There are all kinds of things it could be," Jeff says to me later, as we climb into bed. "Benign tumors. Fatty deposits. We don't really know."

"Absolutely," I reply with a halfhearted smile. Maybe there is a correct way to respond when you get the news that you might—or then again might not—have a potentially fatal recurrence of your cancer, but I don't know what it is. It's kind of like someone pointing a gun at you that might—or then again might not—be loaded. Do you shrug or do you panic? Shrugging seems like a better plan, especially when you know you can always switch to panic later. But had I known then what I know now—that my doctors will soon be calling me in their reports a patient with a "presumptive diagnosis of Stage 4 melanoma" who was getting checked "to establish metastatic disease"—I'd surely have panicked.

August 2, 2011
While Jeff and the girls are spending a long and I hope distracting day at Coney Island with friends, I am sitting in my seersucker gown again as Dr. Partridge makes perfunctory chitchat before getting around to the cancer talk. It's almost exactly one year since the day of my diagnosis, just as bright and pleasant as it was 12 months ago. Where better to celebrate my cancerversary than Sloan Kettering?

"I've reviewed your scans," Dr. Partridge says, "and they're not encouraging. I don't like to wait around with growths. I'm going to recommend you go over to our thoracic department for a consultation about a surgical biopsy. In the meantime we'll do the mutation test on that melanoma we removed last year."

Within this institution full of orchids and free saltines in the waiting area, this place is teeming with cancer. The people who work here are just trying to move it from the bald people sitting outside in the waiting room into dishes and slides and cabinets within. Somewhere in Sloan Kettering, the original tumor that tried to kill me is preserved, like Han Solo in carbonite. "If we need to treat you further," she continues, "I want you to meet with the immunology team again and talk to them."

"I thought the lung nodules were too small to biopsy," I protest.

She gives a thoughtful squint and says, "One of them is pretty deep, in a delicate part of the lung. The other one is close to the surface. I think Dr. Risk can hit it. Once he sees what's going on with that one, we'll know what we're dealing with. It's fairly straightforward. You wouldn't have to stay in the hospital too long."

"His name is Dr. Risk? You think he can hit it?" I ask. This is all very confidence inspiring. Where's Dr. Sure Thing? I'd like to schedule a meeting with him. And I thought biopsies were brief, in-office affairs. I suppose, come to think of it, that taking mystery nodules out of a person's lung is a little more elaborate.

"You're a good candidate for a successful procedure," Dr. Partridge explains. "You're doing well, right? You feel all right? You're young, you're in excellent shape."

I'm 45 and my doctor clearly suspects I have cancer that has metastasized into my lung, but sure, I'll play along. "I guess so," I say. As she gropes purposefully around my lymph nodes, it sinks in that I really might have cancer again. And with that sobering thought, I learn that's how you get through a lymph node check without giggling.

"I'm probably healthier now than I was a year ago," I say. "I'm taking care of myself. Things are good. It's like that phrase I bet you hear all the time, right? I've had the gift of cancer."

She pulls her hands away and shakes her head. "Gift? Oh no," she says. "That's the worst gift I could possibly think of."

In a world in which people who've had cancer are routinely expected to be heroic and inspirational, it is very nice to have a doctor who understands that cancer is actually just a really unpleasant thing to have life hand you.

"Well, I had been hoping for a set of car keys under my seat," I admit, "but I guess this was what I got instead." Now I have to face the very strong possibility that my cancer is the gift that keeps on giving.

When I finish with Dr. Partridge, she sends me to Dr. Risk's office for a brief preliminary surgical consult. Dr. Risk is confident, articulate, and personable. I'm not the sort of person who needs to do loads of investigative reporting on a person before I let him carve me up; instead, I just talk to him a few minutes and think, I'll bet he can hit it.

Then when I finish with Dr. Risk, I go over to the immunology department. Dr. Esposito, who I met with back in the fall, moved on just a few weeks ago to a post in Boston. Now I have been transferred to a colleague named Dr. Jedd Wolchok.

Dr. Wolchok is roughly my age but strikes me as so capable and avuncular I immediately feel like a trusting child in his presence. He is thin and compact, with salt-and-pepper hair and steely blue eyes. In his white lab coat, he almost seems to disappear into the spare examining room. You can tell he's a doctor because he instinctively opens doors with his elbows. Yet there is something about him that reminds me of Steinbeck's description of Doc in *Cannery Row*—a "cool warm" man whose face, like Doc's, tells the truth. "So you're a patient of Dr. Partridge?" he asks as he shakes my hand. "Let's see what we can do for you today. I've been going over your information, and I think if it turns out you need some therapy after the surgery you'd be a good candidate for systemic treatment."

I am keenly aware of the starkness of the entire situation, but his manner is so genial, so pleasant, it's almost old-fashioned. I find it hard to believe he grew up in New York, though he did, right on Staten Island. His mother was a public school teacher in Brooklyn. He went to school downtown at Stuyvesant before landing at

Princeton. And though I may like to joke about Sloan Kettering being my second home, for him, it really is.

Back in 1984, while he was still just a college freshman, Wolchok found himself on a student project at Sloan Kettering, working with cancer immunologists Alan Houghton and Lloyd Old. His task involved observing the blood samples in melanoma patients who were being treated with a synthetic antibody that recognized a target on cancer cells. Antibodies—also known as immunoglobulins—are proteins that recognize and lock on to invaders. Our immune system naturally produces them, but they can also be created outside the body and introduced as a method of fighting disease. Wolchok observed it in action in those patients: Their tumors were going away. The regressions with that earlier form of therapy, unfortunately, didn't last. But as Wolchok says later, "It was very clear to me that this *could* work." He was hooked. That lab he started out in is now the same lab he oversees.

He has also studied music, and plays the tuba in a local ensemble, the Brooklyn Wind Symphony, in his spare time. I will someday ask him why he didn't pursue a career in music, and he will reply in utter seriousness, "Do you know how hard it is to make it as a professional musician?" My musician friends will find this question—and the knowledge that it might just be easier to develop cures for cancer in long-dismissed fields of scientific study than make a go of it in their industry—remarkably validating.

"Dr. Partridge said chemo was a wash for melanoma," I reply, "so I don't understand how this is different."

"The rationale is clear," he explains patiently. "The immune system is there to protect you against dangerous illness. Defining cancer as a dangerous illness is not a big stretch. What this type of treatment does is take the brake off the system to let it go fight the cancer. It makes sense."

"So you believe this works?" I ask him.

He smiles. "Yes. For a long time, there was a lot of skepticism. Then came ipilimumab. We're seeing the evidence now. Immunotherapy," he tells me, "is like religion. For years, we just had to go on faith." He thinks a moment and then adds, "Well, faith and data."

I've been at Memorial since eight in the morning, and it's a lot to get my head around, but I have a team and my team's plan sounds promising, and that's good enough for now.

After my epic marathon of meetings, I walk directly from Sloan Kettering to Grand Central Station and then head out to Westchester, to spend the rest of the day helping Jeff's mom set up her new computer. It's a useful distraction from the fear of an agonizing death thing, and it feels good to be doing something for someone else. It isn't until hours later, when I'm standing languidly on the train platform like a character out of Cheever, waiting for the Metro-North to take me back into the city, that I finally look at my phone.

There's a new voice mail from Deb. "Hey," she begins, and there's an unnerving mechanical hissing in the background. "I'm just calling to see how it went on your big day, and to let you know I'm in the hospital because part of my bowels fell out. So call me, okay?" Just then, as I listen to her voice in the warm light of early evening, the train pulls in, and for a beat I consider the compelling efficiency of leaping in front of it, just to beat cancer at its game.

I don't want to have a conversation about dislodged bowels on the 7:10 to Grand Central, so I endure the ride, my heart racing all the way, until we pull in at 125th Street. As I begin to walk the long stretch toward the A train, I take out my phone and call her back. "Jesus, Deborah Ann, you just had to top me," I say.

"I'm fine," she says, while machines drone behind her. "What's up with you? I thought you had these lung spots for a while. What's the big deal now?"

"They're growing," I tell her. "I'm having surgery to see if it's lung mets."

All she says is a grim "Oh."

"Enough about my day," I reply. "Why is your junk falling out?"

"The Avastin they have me on has been working great," she says. "My numbers are down low again. I feel good. Apparently this is a pretty common side effect."

"Really? Losing your organs? That's a bitch of a side effect," I reply, as a shirtless man tries to sell me a single cigarette.

"There's nothing keeping my insides in," she explains. "I was in the shower this morning and I felt something sliding out of me. I looked at it and it was pink and shiny, and I shoved it back in and called the doctor."

Okay, wow.

"I called my doctor and spoke to the nurse, and she said she thought it might be one of those things that happens when your bladder drops. I guess that occurs a lot. Anyway, I went in to the doctor and told them that something had popped out, and after that they didn't let me stand up again. They drove me around the corner to the hospital in an ambulance.

"Tomorrow they're going to operate," she continues. "They'll take my lower intestines out, and the reconstructive surgeon will rebuild my vagina with a piece of my abdomen. It's risky because I'm not supposed to have surgery right now. The meds interfere with clotting and wound healing. It's considered 'emergency' work, but what am I supposed to do? Who knew what could fall out of you in the shower?" In a lifetime of daily hygiene, I have only ever dropped soap and an occasional bottle of Head & Shoulders, and neither of those slid out of my body, so yeah, this is pretty revelatory.

I cannot believe how calm she sounds. In contrast, I have now had to stop in the doorway of the Taco Bell to take some cleansing, trying-not-to-faint breaths. "Well, good luck," I say, "because I am cringe-walking my way through Harlem right now with a look of horror on my face."

"No, it's cool," she says. "I'm going to have a supervagina. It's a lot of responsibility."

"You'd better be careful," I tell her. "I've seen *Battlestar Galactica,* and those things always turn on their masters." Then I add, "I'll be thinking of you tomorrow. Happy new vagina."

I walk by street merchants with card tables heavy with hats and incense, until I spot a tiny storefront church with a table laid out in front. There's an open book on it with the words "Prayer List" emblazoned at the top. Below are two columns—a list of names and next to them, intentions. So many people. So many prayers. Beneath the last one, I write the word "Debbie." Next to it, I write another word. "Grace."

I call myself a Christian and I pray every day. I am grateful when people say they're praying for me. So why is it, then, that I want to punch a wall when someone suggests that the outcome of my health or anyone else's is dependent upon the whim of God?

I have always been uncomfortable around the concept of a deity who grants rewards to those he deems worthy or punishes those who displease him. That doesn't work for me. I don't believe in a God who sides with one particular football team on any given Sunday any more than I believe in a God who heals some people from cancer because they prayed correctly—but manages to let children and moms and plenty of nice people die of it all the time. I don't want a God who plays favorites. Prayer to me doesn't mean asking for what I want, even if what I want is something perfectly reasonable like not having cancer again or Debbie not dying on the operating table tomorrow. It means being open to connection. I have felt, in a visceral way, the power of prayer and intention and whatever you want to call it. I've felt it as a gesture of love, a love that is both human and divine. It gives me comfort and strength. But when it comes to the literal work of fighting cancer, I'll take doctors and medicine. I have faith in things that science cannot prove. I believe in things it can.

I also reserve the right to blow on dandelions and throw pennies into the fountain at Lincoln Center.

When I come in at night, the kids have already been fed and are in their pajamas and reading on the couch, worn out from their day with Daddy. I wave wanly at them and go into the bedroom, where I assume my regular end-of-day position under the ceiling fan. Jeff slides down in the bed next to me.

"How did it go?" he asks. It's the first chance we've had to talk. This hasn't been the kind of day to relay information over a text, or even a hurried phone call while the kids are screaming in the background.

"I have lots of cancer news coming in, and it's taking a lot out of me," I tell him. "I'm having a surgical lung biopsy. Dr. Partridge all but told me that she thinks the cancer's back and it's metastasized. Then Debbie called to tell me her insides are falling out. She needs surgery. Like the kind that could go seriously wrong. You know the first thing she said when I talked to her? She wanted to know how I was. Christ."

Jeff sighs like some outside force is squeezing all the air out of him. It's a heavy, defeated sound.

"I can't keep trying to figure out how it'll all turn out okay," I say in reply. "I'm so tired of being hopeful. Pessimists don't struggle or ask for miracles. They get knocked down, they stay down. This whole past year, we just keep getting up, and then we get beaten down again and again."

"I guess so," Jeff shrugs, "but at least we get a few more turns being up."

We don't say much else. We just lie there in the cool darkness and listen to the low hum of the fan, steady as a heartbeat.

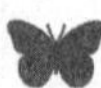

Late the next afternoon, I am drinking iced tea and tapping on my laptop at the Indian Road Café and feeling somewhat catatonic with distraction when Debbie's husband, Mike, calls me. "The surgery went great," he says. "Everything is going to be fine. Oh, except she has to stand on her head from now on." I let out a loud chuckle of relief. She's going to spend the next few weeks recovering, and then she's starting on the chemo drug Abraxane.

"I cannot believe how gangster your wife is," I say, "pushing her internal body parts around and whatnot. I'm pretty sure now that she killed Tupac. Tell her that I love her and I'm thinking of her, and that even though we can't do all our sex stuff, she can still pleasure me." When I talk to her the next day, she sounds groggy but profoundly relieved.

The next weekend we drive down to Washington, D.C., to visit Jeff's high school friends and my cousin Maggie and her daughter, and to show the girls the city for the first time. It's only mid-August, but each moment of the weekend has a deeply wistful, end-of-summer feel. In two weeks, we'll be on Cape Cod. I'll be recovering from my own surgery, and will know for certain if the cancer is back. Maybe it's not. I have to cling to that hope. They're tiny spots. This could all just be something else, something totally minor. That's how we'd explained it to the kids: that the doctors just need to see what's going on. We must have done a good job, because they don't seem terribly concerned at all. They're having fun. That's how I want it. We have long, lazy dinners catching up with family and old pals. We see the Wright brothers' airplane and tour the Capitol. I take the kids to where I stood on the Mall for Obama's Inauguration.

It's just past sundown on Sunday night when we pull in to the Joyce Kilmer rest stop for a turnpike dinner of hot dogs, one last detour before home. By the time we finish, night has fallen completely. As we walk back toward the car through the parking lot, the sight of the New Jersey sky over this dumpy Nathan's Famous strikes me as one of the most profoundly beautiful things I've ever experienced. I remember looking through Jason's telescope that night in March. This is where we come from. This is where we go. I climb into the car and buckle up, and I'm so moved I can barely speak. It's like I've been hit upside the head with the entire cosmos. Just for tonight, I'm at peace with my place in the heavens.

"I had a religious experience somewhere around Exit 9," I tell Jeff later that night. "I was looking up at the stars, and I thought, whatever happens, it's okay. You're part of the universe. You're connected to it forever. It was incredible."

"Yeah, well," he says. "That's nice that you want to go be a star somewhere in the Milky Way. But I just spent five hours in the car with those kids, and there's no way you're leaving me alone with them. You're not going into the light. You're not leaving to become a moonbeam. Forget it. I won't let you. Fuck off." It's the sweetest thing anyone's ever said to me.

It's three days later, and I have been abruptly summoned back to Sloan Kettering. I'm sitting next to an old man curled up under a leopard skin coat when I hear someone call for Mary Williams.

An hour earlier, Dr. Partridge had phoned in the middle of my workday. "Before any procedure like the one you're having, my colleagues and I get together to review all the patients' tests," she had explained. "Last night our radiologist saw something on the soft tissue around your perianal area that we have to check out immediately. Frankly, I was underwhelmed by it, but we need you to come in this afternoon."

Well, I'm sorry my rectal scan underwhelmed you, Doc. My friend Shannon always says that as long as you trust your doctor, the only time you need to freak out is when she says she needs you to come in right away. I guess this is one of those times that Shannon would advise me it'd be okay to freak out. This afternoon, I had hastily finished a movie review, hopped on the subway, and hauled myself back to the hospital, where I now find myself again in seersucker, bracing for a whole lot of anal probing.

Dr. Partridge slowly pulls on her gloves and scours my nether regions with her fingers, checking for moles. She parts the cheeks and looks between them. Then she unceremoniously squirts some lube on her hands and goes in for an incredibly thorough internal exam. As she probes the terrain of my rectum, I wonder if she really needs to do this or she just lost a bet. "You're in good shape," she says. "Nothing unusual. No need to biopsy."

"Thanks," I say. "I appreciate you checking to be sure." I also hate her a little right now for the surprise Wednesday afternoon fisting I've just received.

I start to walk through the bright sunlight from east to west, in the direction of the A train. I never take the crosstown E train. No matter how bad the weather, I always walk. I need that buffer zone between my hospital visits and my regular life. I need to listen to Bruno Mars. And right now, I need to talk to Debbie.

"How's your vagina doing?" I ask. "Can you open beer bottles with it yet?"

"Are you kidding me?" she says. "Pickle jars."

"Well, I can do that with my anus after the exam I've just had," I tell her, as I proceed to unspool the events of my afternoon. I'm expecting some of the jokey Debbie I love to distract me out of the pissed-off mood I cannot seem to shake.

Instead, she says, "I am extremely not okay with this."

I stop walking, right there in the middle of the busy sidewalk on 53rd Street, and I tell her the truth. "I'm extremely not okay too," I admit. "It's all great they can do these miraculous things, and I'm glad they're going over me so carefully. But I am so tired of feeling chipped away. They got part of my head and my hair, they got lymph nodes, they got my thigh. Now they're going to take out part of my lung. I know you can't always go through life with everything you came in with, but I'm starting to feel like the Black Knight from *Holy Grail.* What are they going to lop off next? I'm slowly being robbed of my own body, and I can't even hold a candle to you, Deb—you're basically hollow inside now. You probably rattle when you walk."

"I know," she sighs. "A huge team of people took a piece of my abdomen to rebuild my vagina. My doctor is writing an article on vaginal cuff evisceration, thanks to me. I'm doing okay, but I feel like, how many more times can I get on that table? How many more times can they take something out of me? I want this thing to leave us alone now." I want this to leave us alone too. All of us. Debbie and Mike and Jeff and the girls and Mom. It turns out that after a pop rectal violation, sometimes you just hit the wall.

Two days later, a package arrives. There's no return address and no note. It doesn't need one. Inside is a black T-shirt with the image of an armless, legless, bloody stump of a man. Emblazoned across the front are the words: IT'S JUST A FLESH WOUND.

CHAPTER 13

The Storm

August 25, 2011

The morning of my surgery is muggy and still. It's a quietly menacing sign of the hurricane currently brewing off the Atlantic coast.

This time, Jeff comes with me to the hospital. "It could be a lot of things," he says as we ride downtown. "I'm still going to assume it could be benign. There's no reason not to maintain hope." I pat his hand and stare out the window.

The kids finished up summer camp a few days ago and are already at Jeff's mom's. The plan is that they'll stay with her while I have my procedure, then we'll all meet up at the house and go to the Cape on Saturday, just as we'd originally scheduled it. Jeff and I ride up the elevator together to the same floor I was on a year ago, where the man at the front desk had jokingly told me not to come back. I'm back. Back walking down the hallway to the waiting area, past a row of "consultation rooms" for patients and their families. Each one has tissue boxes scattered conspicuously around. I wonder if this place has a Yelp rating as one of the top buildings in New York City for copious weeping.

When the concierge comes to escort me back to pre-op, he introduces himself politely. "I'm Tom, Ms. Williams. How are you today?"

"White-hot terror and dread, Tom, thanks," I reply.

I know the routine this time, the placing of my clothes in the garment bag, the donning of skid-proof slippers, the uncomprehending gazing at the pages of the new Lev Grossman novel. This is everything I'd feared when I first came here. It's home. A young doctor comes in with a clipboard full of paperwork and asks if I would be willing to donate the tissue they remove from me for a study they're doing of melanoma. I happily sign my tissues over, satisfied at the thought that my evil cells are serving science, and only somewhat paranoid that I'll be responsible for the melanin-fueled clone army that eventually enslaves humanity.

My anesthesiologist Paula, dark haired and surprisingly smoking hot, drops by to ask some questions and check me out. "Open your mouth," she purrs in her Milanese accent, and I unhinge my jaw like I'm trying to swallow a rabbit. "Wide. Wider. Great." I shut my mouth and she looks ridiculously pleased. "You're an anesthesiologist's dream," she says. "You're thin and you have a large mouth." Trust me, I think, in my 20s, that combination didn't just make me popular with anesthesiologists.

An hour later, an orderly comes to escort me to surgery. "I'll see you on the other side," I tell Jeff, and walk once again down the long, cold corridor into the operating theater. It's just a little surgery. It's just two dots in my chest. It doesn't have to be cancer.

I slide onto the table and the doctors cover me with blankets. Paula is there, smiling. I turn my head to see the drip by my arm. There's much bustling now, but I'm calm. I slowly lower my eyelids, and when I open my eyes again I am in post-op. "You're all finished," a faraway voice says. "Here's your button if you need pain management. Jeff will be here soon."

Based on this thick stupor of postsurgical anesthesia and happy dopiness I'm enjoying, Paula must have really gone to town on me. I close my eyes again and open them when I hear the scrape of a chair. Jeff is sitting beside me; one bleary look at his forlorn, weary face and I know. I'll be needing some more reality-obliterating opiates to handle what he's going to say to me now.

After the surgery, Dr. Risk, still clad in his surgical blue scrubs, had come out to where Jeff had been waiting and ushered him into one of those small meeting rooms with the boxes of tissues, and had told him how it had gone and what he had seen. Jeff had sat with him, trying to fathom the enormity of what the surgeon was telling him and to remember it correctly so that he could then turn around and tell it to the mother of his children. Jeff had stood up and said, "Thank you." He had watched me for a while, asleep on a gurney, had seen my eyes flutter open expectantly when he sat down next to me, and he had asked himself how he was going to speak to me without getting upset.

"The procedure went well," Jeff says. "They got the one spot out of your lung, which is great. The doctor says he's 99 percent sure it's malignant. The other was too deep. He's going to talk to the immunology team about drugs to shrink it, and you'll go from there." He tells me it all in a cool, soothing voice.

I am flat on my back as the tears begin to roll down onto my neck. "I'm sorry," I say over and over again. "I am so so so sorry." In all of my fear over the past few weeks, I'd still clung to foolish hope. I'd entertained the fantasy of hearing Dr. Risk tell me it was just some benign growth and, whew, what a crazy scare that was, huh? The truth is that I am such a failure. Such a cause of anxiety in my family's lives. I tried, everybody, I really did. I feel the morphine kick in and dreamily assess the situation. Metastatic melanoma. The optimism of the past few weeks floats away in an opiate fog.

Soon, the nurses roll me into my room, where the bewigged woman in the other bed is currently belting out "Together, Wherever

We Go" from *Gypsy* with assorted family members. "With you for me and me for you, we'll muddle through whatever we do, together!" they sing. Her name is Juliet. She's a cabaret singer. She has lung cancer.

"Are we bothering you?" she asks.

"No," I say sleepily. "I was just wondering if you take requests."

When the nurse brings me lunch—a tray of strawberry Jell-O and broth—I ask if I can get help going to the bathroom. I can barely move on my own yet. There's a drainage tube coming out of my back and an oxygen tube coming out of my nose.

"Not yet," she says. "You've got a catheter. You can get up when we remove it at midnight."

"Midnight?" I ask. "Is that when the catheter fairy comes?"

All afternoon, Jeff sits with me while I drowse uncomfortably and press the round, red button that delivers measured doses of happy juice. Do I, at some point in all of this, talk to the girls? Do I attempt a perky-voiced, "Hi, it's official: Mommy's got more cancer!" conversation or do I leave the bad-news breaking entirely to Jeff? I don't know. Of the many, many traumatic things that have happened in this cancer odyssey of mine—and of all those still yet to come—this is the place my mind goes forever resolutely blank. I remember Juliet and her show tunes. I remember watching *Bring It On* through a narcotic haze. I remember dropping off to sleep and waking up in intense, rapidly amplifying pain, repeatedly. I remember dark clouds rolling in the sky outside. Yet of how my daughters learned that their mother's cancer had returned and metastasized, I have nothing at all. My mind refuses not just to remember it but even to imagine it. I think my mind probably knows what it's doing.

Eventually, after they've polished off the pizzas they have brought in from Patsy's, Juliet's family takes off, and Jeff has to as well. For a few minutes there's no sound in the room except the rhythmic drone of monitors and machines. Then Juliet turns on the Weather Channel. She falls asleep immediately, so I spend the night in and out of narcotic rest, lulled by the escalatingly frantic reports about how Hurricane Irene is galloping ever closer to landfall. We were supposed to go to Cape Cod Saturday. Now the mayor is evacuating parts of the city, and I am here with cancer in my lung. It's a fitful night.

In the morning, Jeff is back at my bedside when Dr. Risk stops by. "The surgery went well," he says. "The other growth is small, and because of its delicate location, we think the best plan for you now is to treat this systemically. There are some very exciting new drugs available now."

"I wasn't really looking for excitement," I say.

He pretends he didn't hear that as he continues. "We're fortunate—ten years ago we probably wouldn't even have been able to find the tumor at this size."

Fortunate me, I have just a speck of malignant, metastatic cancer. "When you come back in a few weeks," he continues, "you and Dr. Partridge will talk more about your course of treatment. In the meantime, you go home and enjoy your vacation." The last time a doctor suggested I go enjoy myself, I wound up getting fisted by my oncologist.

Later, they roll me down to x-ray and park me in the waiting area with the rest of the lung cases. We sit together in our hospital socks and awkwardly tied robes, clicking our buttons when the sensations of our bodies trying to knit themselves back together become too difficult to bear.

It's still early in the day, but the whole floor is buzzing with activity. "They're evacuating NYU Hospital," my nurse tells me. "They're sending oncology patients up here. Anyone who can go home, they're discharging now." I'm doing well and my oxygen levels are stellar, but this new GTFO plan is not the leisurely recuperative day I'd envisioned. The nurse untethers me from my beloved morphine button and hands me release papers, a spirometer to help me exercise my cancery lung and to gauge how successfully I'm breathing, and three bottles of pills: a jumbo portion of Percocet, stool softener, and laxatives. Good times. All we need to do now is get uptown and then out to Mom's. During an exodus.

Once outside, Jeff flags a taxi. Its air conditioner is broken, and the combination of Friday afternoon traffic combined with the Hurricane Irene stampede makes the streets barely passable. My meds are wearing off quickly now, and my freshly operated-on lung is asserting its irritation with the situation. I sit in the backseat, increasingly short of breath in the humid heat and car exhaust. By 145th Street, I'm in wrenching pain and can barely breathe. I suddenly have only one panicky thought now—that I cannot stay in this car a minute longer. So, at a traffic light, I grab the door handle and abruptly jump out. It's possible I'm not thinking too clearly here.

Jeff thrusts a few bills into the driver's hand while I gasp frantically on the sidewalk. I feel like an animal. I cannot even speak; I can only make desperate wheezing sounds. Can't breathe. Can't breathe. Can't breathe. I look helplessly at Jeff while passersby flutter to my side, asking if I need a place to sit down. A grandmotherly woman even offers me a hit off her asthma inhaler. I wave them all off as Jeff guides me into a Starbucks, where I sit in the chilly artificial air, shaking as I try to get my breath back. Jeff manages to procure a small paper bag, the kind they usually slip those nice vanilla scones in, and hands it to me. "Breathe," he says. I'm not sure I remember how.

When I've cooled down and am breathing somewhat regularly again, we get another cab, this time with air-conditioning, and I immediately doze off in the backseat. Even without the hurricane, I don't think a five-hour car ride to Wellfleet tomorrow would have been in the cards. Instead, Jeff, the kids, and I will spend the weekend at Mom's, watching the storm howl around the house while we all remain cozily bunkered inside.

August 27, 2011
"What's this fun little thing?" Lucy asks, turning over my spirometer curiously as I sluggishly try to follow the plot of an old *Friends* episode. It is two days after my surgery.

"I have to blow into it to practice breathing," I reply. "I try to make the blue thing go up as high as I can."

"Ooh, can I play with it too?" Bea asks. They haven't enjoyed any of my cancer apparatus this much since the elf caps.

"Sure," I tell her, "but I know you'd beat me in getting to the highest line."

The time passes like a dream—a narcotics and Sandra Bullock movies on cable TV–fueled dream, where the reverie is only occasionally shattered by the sound of a falling tree or Mom's radio downstairs, full of news reports advising people whether to stay or leave the area. Underneath it all, there's the constant hum of not what's outside but what's inside—the pain where my body was opened and the realization that I do indeed have cancer in my lung. We have to make it to Wellfleet. This may be my last chance.

The kids sense it too. Lucy will later tell me how that weekend, as the wind whipped outside their bedroom, she admitted to Bea, "I'm scared about Mommy." She will tell me that she wanted Bea to know that they could talk about it. She will say that Bea had answered her, "Me too."

On Sunday we sit together at the table after dinner, eating brownies that Mom has made for us. They are extraordinarily child- and person with cancer who might want to eat her feelings-friendly—thickly frosted and covered in round candy sprinkles.

I am wearily biting into mine when Lucy has a question. "I'm confused," she says. "If you had surgery, why do you still have cancer?"

"They got one of my spots out, but the other one was too hard to reach," I explain. "We're probably going to do some treatment to make it go away. Like medicine."

"Well, how much cancer is still in there?" she asks.

"Tiny bit," I say, just like the doctors told me. I pick a round yellow circle off the brownie. It's a little smaller than the space left by a hole puncher. "Like a sprinkle." Just big enough to scare the hell out of me.

By Monday morning, the storm has blown through and left us intact. Although I'm still aching and exhausted, both the weather and my respiration are in promising enough shape to go at last up to the Cape.

But first, now that I've waited more than the required 72 hours since the surgery, I am dying to take off my hospital bandages and take a real shower. "Will you help me?" I ask Jeff as he's tossing toiletries into a bag. Then I slowly peel off my oversize T-shirt and walk toward him in his mother's sunlit guest room, my torso clad only in gauze and tape.

"Tell me if this hurts," he asks, carefully pulling off the largest bandage, directly under my left breast. He looks scared but determined. "I don't want to hurt you." He then moves around to the other side, removing the one on my mid-back. Finally, he takes off the covering over the sorest, meanest wound, right at my left armpit. There are crimson gashes underneath all three sites, all deep and ragged, surrounded by stubborn globs of glue. This was all for a procedure considered minor, for the growth the docs said would be easy to get.

"You look like you've been stabbed," Jeff says.

"You should see the other guy," I tell him.

We have to get on the road in a few minutes, but he just stands there, wordlessly, looking at me. Then he starts to cry. "I am very mad about this," he says.

I fold my right arm around him cautiously, as he sobs into my shoulder.

Then on this brilliant blue morning after the storm, my first Monday as a person with metastatic cancer, we all drive up to Wellfleet—Jeff, Mom, the kids, and me. I spend most of the ride passed out, my head smooshed into a pillow pressed against the window. We ride past entire towns that don't have electricity, past rest stops still shut down. The day is fiercely bright and just a bit cool, like it sometimes is right after a big storm. Like it sometimes is at the close of summer.

It is a strangely great trip. It's good being away for this recovery time. Much of it feels easy and comfortable, and the rest of it is like being on an entirely different planet. We eat corn on the cob and splash in Gull Pond and play miniature golf at Poit's. I only go up to my waist in the water this time, though, to protect my surgical wounds, and my putt-putt game is far from my best. I spend many of my hours napping and reading and trying to resume physical activity while Jeff and Mom attend to the cooking and laundry and having coherent conversations. Sometimes I watch Jeff and the children as I sit weakly nearby, and think what an unexpected present our marital estrangement turned out to be. Jeff's always been a good dad. I know from experience that he's also a good single dad. He knows how to take care of those kids on his own. That's a training that may well come in handy for him again soon.

In the moments I am not fending off an assload of pain, I feel like I'm floating outside of it all, observing myself blowing into the spirometer, putting together jigsaw puzzles with calm detachment, drifting to sleep at the drive-in before the opening credits of the latest installment of the Spy Kids franchise are even over. I chalk it up to a combination of coming off the anesthesia, the Percocet I am on, and the not-to-be-underestimated shock that I really do have more cancer. Every night, the sun goes down a few minutes earlier, and our sweatshirts come on a little sooner. It all feels achingly bittersweet. This must be how Dad felt, when he said Christmas was really over. In my photos from the trip, I have a faraway look in my eyes and a belly bloated from narcotic constipation.

On our penultimate night, we are finishing up our evening ice-cream cones outside of Mac's when we hear the sound of some old-school disco emanating from the farthest end of the pier. It's an informal dance party, with a DJ and grown-ups and kids and teenagers swaying in the crisp early September air to KC and the Sunshine Band and the Bee Gees. The girls run instinctively in the direction of the music. I am tired. I am hurting. It's been a long day, and I am just about ready for a painkiller. "You go ahead," I tell Jeff. "Mom and I will catch up."

Summer is ending. My brief time as a cancer success story is over. But, hey, they're playing the Village People, and if I'm on my way out, I'm going out like a leather man or a cowboy or an Indian chief. I can do this. I want to do this. I want to dance with my family. I break into a run and find my place between Jeff and the girls. It's worth it to watch my daughters laugh under the moon near a harbor. Because maybe next summer they'll be dancing without me. Though it hurts to lift my hands above my head, I know you cannot spell YMCA without the Y. And if my obituary reads, "Ridiculous woman dies overdoing it to seventies grooves," that will be just fine with me.

CHAPTER 14

Stage 4

September 2011

By the time I go for my postsurgery checkup, fall has already fully descended. Lucy has started at her new middle school, and we are cobbling together a clumsy schedule for getting her all the way downtown in the morning and all the way back uptown in the afternoon. She's settling in well so far, though her new routine is exhausting for all of us. Bea, meanwhile, is relishing her new status as a hot-shit second grader and the sole member of the family at her elementary school.

Though I am a bit of a basket case, Dr. Risk is chipper and breezy. "The melanoma that traveled to your lung likely did so before your operation last year, which would mean no new growth," he says.

This is a massive relief, an assurance that in spite of the setback, everything is under control. "We'll see how the drugs do, but in the meantime it looks like you're healing well and getting back on track."

Less than a month ago, the FDA approved another new melanoma drug—Genentech's vemurafenib, also known as Zelboraf, for patients who possess a particular mutation in their BRAF gene. Roughly half of all people with melanomas have it. Mine does not, so I don't qualify for the drug. Instead, Dr. Partridge is interested in putting me on a course of that much buzzed about new drug ipilimumab, the one the FDA approved last March. My new immunologist Dr. Wolchok played a leading role in one of the patient trials that led to its approval. I think that ipilimumab, known to doctors by the casual nickname ipi, sounds like a name you'd give a Teletubby, or the national dish of North Korea, or a vengeful Egyptian pharaoh.

"That all sounds good," I say. "While we're here, can you look at this thing on my back?" I hike up my gown, to what looks like a small bruise. It's a distinct, purple line, slightly raised and tender to the touch. I'd noticed it only earlier this week, and surmised it was a mark from the surgery or getting moved around afterward.

He doesn't look surprised or troubled. We both know he and Dr. Partridge have gone over every inch of me, and recently. He just says, "We'd better biopsy you, to be safe. Want to check everything out before the treatment." My consultation report will note that a biopsy was sent to cytology "to confirm that this is not related to any underlying malignancy." Dr. Risk sticks a needle in my back and a bandage over it, and I put my clothes back on and go outside and get a turkey burger and a beer—okay, two beers—for lunch. Less than 24 hours later, a nurse I've never met or spoken to before calls with the results.

"Ms. Williams, your biopsy came back malignant," she says as crisply as if she were confirming an appointment. When you've got cancer, you get one delicate, sensitive phone call—the first one. The rest are pretty straightforward communications of the facts before the person on the other end of the line goes back to eating lunch.

I hang there on the other end of the line, dead silent.

"Are you there?" she says.

"Yes," I say, almost inaudibly. "So am I going to have another operation?"

"We're sending the results to your doctors," she tells me. "They'll discuss with you the best options for a person at Stage 4." Stage 4. Well, that's the first time anybody's said that to me. That's a game changer, what with there being no Stage 5 and all. I suppose I should have figured it out when the cancer moved into my lungs, but I didn't connect the dots. I didn't want to. I still don't reply.

"Where are you right now?" she asks.

"Home," I say.

"Do you have someone you can call and talk to?"

"Yes," I say. Then I hang up and get on with the business of flipping out. I can barely get the words out when I call Jeff. I open my mouth to speak, and deep, choking sobs come out instead. He knows what it means, and he says, "I'll be right home."

When I've pulled myself a little more together, I send an email to a select handful of friends. The subject head is "Cancer continues to be an asshole."

Within minutes, the phone is ringing.

"I want you to know you're a warrior," Debbie declares when I pick up the phone. "So you go, girl." Then she adds, "I'm just kidding. This sucks." That's the Debbie I know and love. "You feel however you want to feel," she says, "because right now I'm going for rage and feeling really sorry for us."

"That sounds perfect," I tell her. "I'm going for shock and tons of fear."

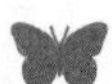

An hour later Jeff and I are sitting at the bar of the Indian Road Café. We don't talk a lot; we just share the space in quiet defeat. What I am thinking, however, is how much I hate the word "survivor." It's a lie. It's a crass fiction that other people impose on you to make themselves feel safe. Like we can all move on now and forget about the cancer. But you cannot forget about cancer. It huffs and it puffs and it blows through your life, and even if it doesn't tear your house down today, it's just going to try again tomorrow. Maybe I'm just a mite fatalistic right now, I think, as I stare into the ruby bottom of a glass of Malbec, because I am such a bad survivor. Because I have cancer. Again. Worse. A lot worse. Dammit, T cells, YOU HAD ONE JOB.

I feel like me. I look, except for all the new scars of the past year, like me. Dr. Risk had said there was likely no new growth, and new growth was blazing up in my body after all. How can I be this sick? How can it be this bad? Is it possible my respected doctor doesn't know anything? My cancer is becoming more insistent. It's going to be a race against time from here on in. So let's start racing.

I am halfway through my second glass of wine when Jeff looks at his watch. "If we settle up now, I figure we have 15 minutes for life-affirming sex before we have to pick up the kids from school."

I cast a sideways glance at him. And I knock back the rest of my glass and motion to the bartender.

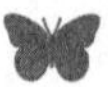

When I go in to see Dr. Partridge, she's considerably more relaxed than I am. "How are you?" she asks casually.

I'm devastated. I'm terrified I won't see my children grow up. I'm dreading the possibility of winding up in a hospice, watching my insides drain into a carafe while I slip in and out of lucid consciousness. I can't think straight because in just a few days, the lump has become more tender and sore, and when I shift in my sleep or put on my shirt, it feels like a giant zit that wants desperately to pop. I'm so freaked out I want to throw up.

"I'm surprised," I say. "I didn't think it would come raging back like this, not after a year."

She gives me a sad, small shrug. "The odds were against you from the start," she says. "We knew that, because of the size and the depth of the melanoma, because of the location, on your head." But you told me I was cancer free, I think. I thought that meant I could stay that way.

When my friend Michele was a lifeguard, beachgoers used to ask her all the time, "Are there sharks in the ocean today?" She'd tell them, "There are sharks in the ocean every day." The cancer has always been a threat. Today, it is swimming up to me. I guess the fact that I've lived this long without getting attacked again is supposed to be encouraging. It's not.

"I've read about this ipilimumab," I say. "I read that people on it lived a median of ten months. And that it worked long-term on only about 20 percent of the patients."

"With your cancer," she says, "that's considered a home run," which makes me glad she's in the oncology business and not the birth control one. I can take the drug with the low chance of success, or the cancer with a considerably higher chance of killing me within a year. The math here is agonizingly simple.

"What about this new tumor on my back?" I ask.

"It just means you have a soft tissue metastasis. It's a subcutaneous tumor." Subcutaneous. Under the skin. "The new tumor doesn't change how we're proceeding with your treatment," she continues, "but, no, I don't like that you have a new melanoma. The rapidity of this makes me anxious, but it confirms our plan to treat you systemically. There's no reason to think this won't work. We'll get you on the ipi, but there's also a very promising trial Dr. Wolchok has been running I'd like to see you in."

The trial, she explains, is the ipi in combination with another Bristol-Myers Squibb drug, so new and mysterious it doesn't even have a name yet. It's just known as MDX-1106. It works in a manner similar to ipi in that it's another monoclonal antibody, one that targets a protein called programmed cell death 1, or PD-1. Like

CTLA-4, PD-1 is a protein that hangs out on the surface of T cells. If another protein, called PD-L1, binds to it, it can thwart the T cells from doing their work. The hope is that the MDX-1106 can run interference, blocking the PD-L1 from getting to its destination and leaving the T cells to do their job.

The trial so far is still only in Phase 1. As the name implies, Phase 1 is the initial stage of a clinical trial for a treatment or combination of treatments. Because the researchers are usually trying the protocol on humans for the first time, they typically take only a small number of patients, who are divided into dose escalation groups to establish safety and efficacy. The earlier the cohort of the trial, the lower the dose usually is. This new trial has only a handful of people in it so far and has been acquiring them selectively. There's one new spot currently earmarked for a patient coming in from the Midwest to do it. "That may fall through," Dr. Partridge tells me, "and then you'd be next in line." As Jedd Wolchok will later explain it to me in terms that are equal parts reassuring and chilling, "For a study like this, which was considered very high risk, the time in between patients was very long, because we did not want to make the mistake of exposing a lot of people at the same time to a toxic regimen," he says. "We wanted to be sure that every single patient that we treated was reasonably safe before exposing another person to that treatment."

Because I am now considerably worse off than I was a year ago when I met with Dr. Esposito, I have been ushered into the VIP room of cancer, a club whose qualifications are a Stage 3 or 4 diagnosis. The rewards are a broader range of clinical trial options. I am fortunate to be getting a fatal form of cancer right at a moment that I have the possibility of jumping into a trial like this.

With new drugs and new protocols, there are inevitable risks. In the clinical study report for ipilimumab, "Adverse events with an outcome of death were reported for 44 subjects, of which 14 were judged by the Investigator to be related to study drug." That's still a small number of people from what was a large and long study, and half of those 14 deaths were judged to be tied to "immune-related adverse events." Still, there's nothing like the words "bowel perforation and liver failure" to give one a case of the willies.

I am nonetheless intrigued at the idea of getting two cancer-fighting drugs instead of one, which certainly seems to better my odds exponentially. I also like that I could be monitored constantly and intensely, which is exactly the amount of attention I'd like right now. You can't fall off the radar if you're a subject of research.

But I am also concerned about why Dr. Partridge is talking to me about a clinical trial. A trial to me implies that she's giving up. I feel like maybe she's throwing in the towel on her failed patient, and preemptively donating my body to science.

"You're very early Stage 4," she says, "and believe me, Stage 4 isn't what it used to be. I believe your long-term prognosis is excellent." That's just swell. Stage 4—it's the new Stage 2! Except it's not. Not really. It's great that medical advancements are giving more people more time, but Stage 4 is not a place people generally come back from. It's usually instead the next to last stop on the Cancer Train before Boot Hill, and everybody knows it. "You're not in pain, you're not symptomatic. Right?" Dr. Partridge asks. I'm not. I will hear these questions again many times in the weeks that immediately follow this conversation. I will learn that when you're Stage 4, doctors ask you a lot if you're in pain. There's a kind of implied inevitability to the inquiry.

"If it's not so horrible, then why aren't you guys just cutting out the tumors in my lung and my back?" I say.

"The one in your lung is in a difficult spot. And we can take the one off your back," she explains, "but the cancer would still be moving around your body. That's why I recommend we try to get you into this trial. The only reason we'd remove a subdermal like that at Stage 4 is for the patient's comfort anyway." I'm sure she means it kindly, but that "comfort" line sounds palliative as hell.

"We'd just be putting out fires," I say quietly. There's not much point.

Dr. Partridge looks at me with a tender gleam in her eye. "It's a simple procedure if you want the back tumor removed. You'll be in and out in a half hour. Let's do it. I think it'll ease your mind."

"There's nothing we can do," I say.

"There's almost always something we can do," she replies, and she means something far more complex than containing cancer. It's about finding some measure of control in an utterly out-of-control situation. It's about not being helpless.

"Okay, then," I say. "Let Dr. Wolchok's team know I'm interested in getting on the list for the trial."

I guess this means we are slowly forming a plan, my cancer team and me, albeit one that may keep changing. Do the ipi. Get the tumor excised. Try to get into the trial. Take it one step at a time. Remember that I am getting lots and lots of help. Try not to hate myself for what's happening to me.

As I get on the A train heading home, I spy a young man in a black T-shirt getting off. His chest bears a message from the movie *Pi*—FAITH IN CHAOS. I stand there on the platform, rooted, staring at him, as the doors close. I'm trying, universe. I'm really trying.

But in addition to keeping the faith, you know what else you have to do when you find out you have Stage 4 cancer? You have to do your laundry. You have to buy the groceries. You have to do your job.

You have to make sure the kids brush their teeth. You have to clean up and do it all over again the next day that you are just trying to stay around for. The world doesn't grind to a halt just because your life might.

"Mom's had a really rough day," I tell the girls as we walk down Broadway heading homeward from their now dual school pickup, before the daily deluge of homework and cooking and baths. They exchange worried looks at each other and grip hands together. "And I think that calls for a little pampering." I lead us up a narrow flight of stairs to the Dominican salon, the one over the pawnshop, to get our hair done. Nearly six years into living in the neighborhood, and I still conduct all my business there with a bright *"Hola! Que pasa?"* followed by a gesture that mimics either the snipping of scissors or the waving of a hair dryer. Why haven't I ever learned Spanish? What was I waiting for? Now I have stupid cancer and I never even got to learn Spanish.

I am nevertheless feeling the most relaxed I've been in weeks as the girls and I sit in our swivel chairs, waving at each other in the mirrors through a thick mist of hair spray. Sure, I've got brand-new cancer popping up in my body, but what's left of my hair is going to look very pretty. Then Lucy's lady comes over and exchanges a few rapid-fire words with my lady, and I can tell from her tone that this day is not yet finished being crappy.

She speaks only a smattering of English, but the word she lobs at me today is potent. "Lice," she says, pointing at Lucy's hair.

"That's dandruff," I say, confident of our family legacy of flaky scalp.

"Lice," she repeats firmly. She looks over at Bea, who's looking fretful but regal in the chair next to her sister. "I think, the baby too." Bea promptly bursts into tears.

We settle up quickly and hustle out the door, our hair still slightly damp, burning with shame at the accusation that we're the lice family. The girls are both sobbing now.

"I swear it's not lice," I insist repeatedly, as they mope and cry all the way home. "I will check you thoroughly when we get to the apartment."

As soon as we walk in and hang up our sweaters, I do just that. I turn on the bright overhead light and sit the girls at the dinner table, don my glasses, and inspect them both. My kids have never had lice. They have dry scalps and get itchy sometimes, but they haven't been clawing their heads lately or anything. I gingerly pull Lucy's hair apart at the crown of her head. There, glistening in her thick tangles of waves, are tiny, glistening, not-to-be-argued-with nits. Then I repeat the process, with the same results, on Bea.

Lucy is inconsolable. "I have lice," she sobs. This day is the goddamn worst.

Now the work begins. I gather up laundry and toss out old hats, and assign the girls the job of pulling their toys off the shelves and their beds and putting them in tightly sealed garbage bags.

When I check in on them in their bedroom a short time later to gauge their progress, Bea is standing mutely in the midst of the mess, holding a small stuffed animal and crying. "It's just for a little while," I say.

"I know," she says. "It's just, I got this one with Grandpa."

It's the unicorn he gave her for her birthday. The last time he saw her.

"He asked me what I was going to name him, and I said that it was a girl, remember?"

"Yeah," I say. We sit together on the edge of her bottom bunk, Bea snuffling softly. "You miss him. It hurts that you miss him, but it's good that you loved him, so you just let it out. It's a lot for a little girl."

She smiles through her tears, like she always does. She grasps my hand, and though I think I'm trying to comfort her, she looks up at me and says the most generous words of comfort to me. "It's okay," she says. "It'll be okay. We'll get rid of the lice. And you're going to be cancer free again too, Mama." Then I'm the one who's crying.

By the time Jeff comes home, he is greeted by a trio of semi-hysterical, vermin-riddled females, and he and I set about the grim task of inspecting each other's heads for bugs like intimate gorilla mates in a nature special. He has miraculously managed to avoid getting even a single nit, but when he checks my scalp, it's obvious I'm infested too. Man, the repulsive things that happen on my head.

The next day the kids have to stay home from school, so Jeff takes a day off from work, because I have to go in to meet with Dr. Wolchok to begin the preliminary exams for my course of ipi. With my hair pulled back in a very tight bun, I have my weight measured and my treatment schedule discussed because I have metastatic cancer, and I am now also trying not to touch my head because it's crawling with bugs. It's a lengthy, stressful morning, so when my friend Joey texts me, "What are you doing right now? Because the answer is, letting Steve and me buy you a drink," I am all over it. I am woozy with emotion and blood loss. A drink sounds about right.

Joey is an advertising executive, married to a roller derby girl, and Steve is a researcher friend from my years in San Francisco, in town on business for his biotech firm.

I arrive at the French restaurant in a sleeveless red dress, freshly exsanguinated and sporting a large bandage on my arm. "Nice bid for sympathy," Steve says. "By the way," he adds, opening his arms for an embrace, "you look beautiful."

"I have lice," I reply, and he deftly shifts course for a fraternal pat on the shoulder. "I have lice and I have Stage 4 cancer."

"And you are," he answers diplomatically, "the most beautiful woman with lice and Stage 4 cancer I have ever seen. So how are you feeling?"

"Like I'm on the real *Wheel of Fortune,*" I say. "Like I could land on 'It'll Be Okay,' or 'Start Making Final Arrangements.' But I guess

I can't complain," I continue, launching into a litany of nervous happy talk. "Everybody at Memorial is great. They're amazing. I'm lucky. Everybody says I'm lucky."

Joey looks at me, amused. "I'm giving you five more minutes," he says, "and then I want you to knock it off with how awesome your cancer is."

"Thank you," I say, "because I'm scared. I'm scared and I have lice."

In search of some measure of intellectual grasp on my increasingly chaotic situation, I ask Steve for some inside dish on Yervoy—and about the combination trial I'm currently wait-listed for. Joey, meanwhile, is tasked with the pressing matter of getting us a minimum of one bottle of wine, ASAP.

"The anti-CTL-4 has already had some very interesting results in monotherapy," Steve says, "and there's an awful lot of excitement around the early research with this other anti-PD-1." This is fancy-science-guy talk for saying that Yervoy, by itself, seems to do the job for some people, and the new drug looks good too. But the kicker—the thing even I understand—is when he says, "These kinds of treatments tend to be superexpensive, and using them in combination is almost unheard of. If I were you, I would try to get in this trial and stay on it as long as I could possibly tolerate it. If you get in, do everything you can to not drop out. If you quit, you're going to have trouble getting in another trial. In the meantime, you're getting an unbelievable deal here. For the cost of the drugs, your net gain on this would be extraordinary." Assuming, of course, that it works.

I'm still having a hard time grasping the science of it all, but I am great at sniffing out a bargain. More than that, though, I can tell from Steve's enthusiasm that he wants this for me. He knows all too well that my very few other treatment options offer slim chance of survival.

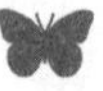

On Saturday, Jennifer, a woman known to uptown parents as the resident local lice guru, comes over. Normally Jeff and I would have tried to suck it up and handle the crisis on our own with some hastily purchased products from Rite Aid, but this has been a pretty outside-the-box week—and Jeff and I feel that if ever there was a problem that needed us to throw a little money at it, this would be the one.

"Before you do the girls," I tell Jennifer, "I need to explain a few things about my condition. I have cancer and I have a skin graft on my head. The graft's over a year old and it's solid, but you just need to be gentle around the edges."

She looks unhappy. "Let me see," she says, and as I bend my head forward and part my hair, she continues. "I don't know. I've never done a job like that."

"It's fine," I repeat. "You just have to be gentle at the edges of the graft." She continues to look unhappy as she sets to work.

Jennifer combs through the girls' hair while simultaneously maintaining a constant level of cell phone chatter. She first turns her attention to Lucy and her tremendous mane of thick curls, and then moves on to Bea and her long, straight tresses. The girls sit patiently on dining room chairs parked in front of the TV the whole time, enjoying an epic binge of the High School Musical trilogy. Jeff and I, in the meantime, run back and forth to hog up the laundry room with the most recently used sheets and clothes.

I am walking in the door with a pile of fresh from the piping-hot dryer towels and Gabriela is joining Troy for a conflict-resolving duet when I notice that Jennifer is nowhere to be seen. Jeff, meanwhile, is looking at me like he does when he has to tell me I have cancer. "She left," he says. "She said she didn't think she could do you."

This is a woman who combs bugs out of children's hair for a living, but my head was too much. She couldn't even face me to tell me. She waited till I was gone for a few minutes to run away. My stupid disfigured head. I feel ashamed, and I'd be full of rage if I wasn't busy being completely defeated. The coward couldn't even say to my face she was leaving. "I'm such a mess," I say, sobbing. "I'm disgusting."

Bea pats my hand gently. "I feel sad for you," she says, plainly.

"It's, okay, Bea; Mom's just feeling her feelings again," says Lucy. I have spent most of my children's lives trying to be strong and reassuring for them. Lately all I do is fall apart in front of them. I've always told them it's okay to cry, but I never set them up for Mama to be the crying one. I don't know how to protect them from this.

"It's not a big deal," Jeff says. "I watched her do the kids. I'm going to go out right now and buy a big bottle of Pantene and a special comb, and Tania can go screw herself."

"Her name is Jennifer," I say.

"And Jennifer," he replies, "can go screw herself."

We spend the rest of the weekend doing impossible amounts of laundry, dragging fine-tooth combs through each other's hair, and smothering bugs under shower caps and mayo. I had thought March was going to take the prize for crappiest month of the year, but wake me up when September ends. For our efforts, the kids will henceforth have a violent aversion to Hellmann's, permanently eradicating tuna fish salad from our lunch repertoire.

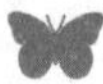

On Monday, Lucy's new school has a meet-and-greet party for the families of the sixth graders and their teachers. I am indifferently regarding a fruit plate—lately my appetite, the one thing in my life that has never failed me, has all but disappeared—when I hear a "Mary Elizabeth? Is that you?" from down the hallway. It's a mom from our old school back in Brooklyn. Her son and my daughter are now, once again, classmates.

"It's been forever!" she says. "How are you? How come you don't keep up your personal blog anymore? You hardly ever update it."

"Yeah," I reply, "things have been busy."

She regards me skeptically. "Busy? Like how?" she demands.

"Well, I have my work and the kids," I say—and then I decide, Let's just get it over with, so I add, "Also, I have cancer."

She blinks. She cocks her head warily. Then she says, "I didn't know you're a survivor."

"I'm not," I reply. "I have cancer."

Her face drops. Perhaps she's flummoxed by the awkwardness of her assumption, but whatever the cause, there's a clear "Get me out of here" expression on her countenance. "Oh," she says. "Well, good luck." With that, she walks quickly away, melting into the crowd of healthier adults and children. As I watch her disappear, I feel broken and useless, like a battered umbrella to be tossed in the trash. Stage 4 may not be what it used to be, but I'll tell you this much—it's still a very small, very lonely club.

CHAPTER 15

Lab Rat

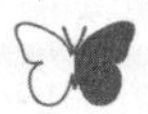

September 2011

It is now getting very bad, and it's happening very quickly. I feel like hell. I suppose it means that I'm dying. It could just be anxiety, but if anxiety means that a person cannot keep any food or liquid in her body, it's still a problem.

My digestive system has now gone on a full strike, refusing to accept even a glass of water without vengefully hurling it back out. I'll be at my desk working, and I'll nibble a bite of toast, trying to quell the urgent hunger. A half hour later I'll feel the cramping in my gut, like a fist in there squeezing it. I'll run to the bathroom again, and make it just in time. I am consequently weak and woozy, my stomach growling demands to be sated, the other parts furiously vomiting and crapping out everything I try to get down. It's what happened to Dad, at the end. His body no longer accepted sustenance. I remember the swampy carafe of his fluids draining by his bedside, and wonder if my body is now eating away at itself too. This is how it starts, I think, exhausted by the dual demands my body is making to fill and evacuate as undigested bits of food stream out of me. Then I clean myself up and go pick up the kids from school.

I'm supposed to start on the Yervoy next week. How will I get through it, when I'm falling apart before it even starts? I am hurtling into the darkness. I never call the doctor, because what if I go to the hospital and I never come home? I'm scared not just of dying—although that certainly is not a ride I'm ready to take—but of what happens when I'm dead. I'm a parent, a partner, and a provider. I care for the kids; I pay half the mortgage. Take me out of the picture and there is an emotional and, frankly, financial, void. I'm imagining Jeff and the kids plunged into economic chaos as well as grief. They'd have to move. Maybe get a cheap rental on the other side of Broadway. Or sell the apartment and move in with Jeff's mom. Damn, and in this market. I'd be the lucky one. I'd just have to die. They'd be stuck with this mess I'd leave behind.

As the days count down to the start of my new treatment, I do my yoga and my meditation. I try so hard to let it all go. Then I panic and I stagger to the bathroom again. I just want to stay, I think as I toss fitfully in bed. I want to stay. I don't want to leave my children, not yet. I say it to myself a million times, over and over and over, like the drunk who won't leave the party. I want to stay. Don't make me leave. Not now, not yet. The school year has barely started and I'm scared I won't see the end of it. Will I see the cherry blossoms in the Botanic Garden in the spring? Will I get to Christmas? Will I make it even to my birthday? Everything I ever thought about the futility of treatments that might only give people who have a fatal disease just a few more months anyway—everything I believed about the pointlessness of it—right now, I take it back. I may well have only a few months, but I want those few months very much. If I could do something to get a few more months on top of that, I'd like to take them too.

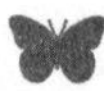

It's early evening when the doorbell rings. I haven't even started making dinner yet, a dinner I strongly doubt I will be able to digest a morsel of. When I open the door, it's the two little girls from down the hall who go to school with Bea, and our three other neighbor kids from down the street. They're holding a tall chocolate cake. Spelled out on it, in white candy stars, are the words "FUCK CANCER."

"Our moms made you something," Natalie, age six, explains. "It has a bad word on it."

"Sometimes in life," I say, "you need a bad word." Then I turn toward Lucy and Bea, doing their homework at the dinner table and say, "Kids, get the plates."

Within a few minutes, the children's parents show up bearing ice cream, sprinkles, syrup, and Reddi-wip. "I told Natalie," her mother, Kristin, explains, "that it was okay to use the bad word because it would make you smile."

"It does," I say. "I'm impressed with both the sentiment and the kerning."

By the time Jeff walks in the door, we have already doled out many slices of cake and scoops of ice cream. I hold my plate and pose for photos, but I can barely get in a bite. If there was a symbolic conquest to be made via consumption of the chocolate cancer cake, I have failed. But if this was a reminder that our family is not alone in this whole miserable thing, then tonight, we've all succeeded quite mightily.

On the Tuesday before I'm supposed to have my first ipi treatment, Dr. Wolchok's office calls. "There's a new spot in the trial," he tells me. "Are you still interested?" I wonder if this means the trial is expanding, or if someone has dropped out or not qualified, or perhaps even, miraculously, gotten better. I hate to consider the other possibility of why that spot has so abruptly become available. My nurse Karen will later speculate, "It could mean we had decided to expand the trial for your dose. It could be somebody's screening failed. It could be they were in the process of eligibility and then they didn't qualify. We had to look at patients based on how well or how sick they were. A clinical trial—it is a lot of responsibility for the patient. And unfortunately, for the very sick," she adds, "this is not always the best avenue for them to take." Fortunately for me, it looks like I am just sick enough.

"I think I am still interested," I say. "Let's say yes?" But now that I have the option of really doing this, I question whether I ought to. I'm cautiously optimistic about the ipi, but know next to nothing about the other drug or its effectiveness and potential consequences. And my consent to doing the trial means not starting immediately on the previously planned single ipi treatment—a nerve-racking delay in getting medicine into me while I'm still playing beat the clock with my fast-acting cancer cells. I remember Steve's encouraging words, but I cannot forget that in most of the movies and television shows I've ever seen, trials are scary. Trials are what you do when you've given up on real medicine. One step above copper bracelets and cannabis oil. What if they give me this weird new drug and it doesn't work, or it makes me even sicker but I've signed off on being a test subject so I'm stuck with it? What if my cancer gets a lot worse while I'm waiting to start the trial? What if I don't even get the drugs? That happens, right? Isn't the whole point of trials that some people get the real drugs and some people get empty useless pills that do nothing?

I say something quite like this, in one big torrent of skepticism and paranoia, when I come back to Memorial for yet another meeting.

Dr. Wolchok is a good doctor because he doesn't look at me like I'm being irrational. He looks at me like he can help. "First of all," he says, "most trials don't involve placebos. That's usually only in later phases. Second, even in those kinds of trials we continue to treat patients. It's not like they're getting nothing; they get the standard of care. Finally, if the trial is not working for someone, or the patient doesn't want to continue for any reason, we can stop at any time and switch to conventional treatment."

I am feeling reassured. A little excited. Hopeful, even. These people don't see me as just an experiment. They want to treat me, as a patient.

Only about 3 percent of eligible adults with cancer participate in clinical trials, and 40 percent of trials never attain their minimum enrollment. Who wants some medical Russian roulette when there are FDA-approved options out there? I am scared too. But for me, the choice is clear. The melanin-producing cells in my body are incredibly resilient. They were designed to be mobile and adaptable—that's why they let me freckle in the summer sun. That's why melanoma tends to fend off chemo and radiation like King Kong swatting biplanes. I don't have time to wait for the new mystery drug to make it safely to the general market, and I don't have a whole lot of other options. And there's something else—the most important and reassuring thing of all. My doctors think this combination has a realistic shot at working on me. As Dr. Wolchok tells me, "This isn't a last course of action. It's a first one."

But before I get started, I have to prove myself truly worthy. Being asked if you'd like to be in a clinical trial is like being accepted into Harvard—you still have to be able to pay for it. The difference here is I don't have to write a check; I just have to submit to a battery of pretrial tests. I need to hit the sweet spot of being sufficiently diseased for the doctors to have something to work with and measure, and healthy enough to withstand whatever it is they're about to unleash on my system. I will later learn, when I read the trial results, that part of my qualifications include having "adequate organ function" and "a life expectancy of at least four months," so I've got that going for me, which is nice. It's funny the things that become your standards of victory when you've got Stage 4 cancer. When I read a medical report that describes my pelvic organs as "unremarkable," I recall, there was probably a time I would have considered that a tad unflattering. When I see that one of the doctors on the immunology team has described me, after a routine consult, as a "well-developed, well-nourished female in no apparent distress," I think it sounds a little like he's describing a cow or a goat he's thinking of purchasing. But I'm eminently glad of it nonetheless.

"All right, then," I say. "Let's do this."

"Let's do this," Dr. Wolchok affirms. "We'll get you started on the next part of the process next week."

That night, I sleep more soundly than I have since that random nurse told me I was Stage 4. I am bug free, and if I pass all the screening tests, I could be getting two superexpensive cancer drugs free, courtesy of medical research. Because it's a trial, Bristol-Myers Squibb would be footing the bill. My regular doctor visits and tests would still be the responsibility of my insurance and me. But all aspects of the treatment itself would be on them. This is better than Groupon. The next morning, I sip some water and down a few spoonfuls of yogurt, and nothing violent happens in my body. Maybe I'll live after all.

INTERLUDE

How to Make a Drug

Though it's gained an unprecedented degree of cachet recently, it hasn't been so long since immunotherapy was a supertough sell. It was hard just to explain. *A lot of people assume that treating cancer means chemo and/or radiation. I've certainly fended off the questions myself, from well-meaning, small talk–making friends and relations. How was your chemo? When do you start chemo? It's chemo, right? Immunotherapy is not chemo. Yes, there's an infusion involved, but not everything dispensed in an IV bag with a "High Alert" warning is chemo. And not getting chemo doesn't mean you didn't have real or serious cancer.*

It's not just laypeople who cannot always get out of chemo as default mode, either. When I later ask Dr. James Allison about his experience as a researcher, he says, "The subtlety of immunotherapy is in the whole paradigm shift. You're not treating the tumor; you're treating the immune system. That's one of the reasons I moved to Sloan Kettering; they understood that."

And a good place to start looking at immunotherapy happens to be with melanoma. As Jedd Wolchok explains, "Melanoma gave us a window into the fact that the immune system might have a role in controlling cancer, because everything is not uniform in melanoma. It can break off, but it can spontaneously regress. If you cast aside divine intervention, the best explanation for spontaneous regression is an immune response to the tumor. That, for a long time, was one of the pillars of support for why immunologists studied melanoma. The other was that the other treatments that were showing efficacy—chemotherapy, radiation—for other kinds of cancer were not so effective in melanoma. It was a strong call for thinking of something creative."

CTLA-4 was first identified by researchers in France back in 1987. But it was Dr. Allison and his team, working in Berkeley, who first figured out that CTLA-4 operates on the T cell as an inhibitor, and theorized that controlling it could hold a crucial key to giving the immune system a fighting chance. It was the beginning of what would become ipilimumab.

"Everything at the time was concentrated on turning T cells on,*" Allison will tell me later, understatedly reminiscing. "I kind of dabbled around. We finally figured out we could, in a very programmed way, turn the brakes* off. *It's kind of like a gas pedal. It's not really that complicated—just suspend the brakes in a way you can control. The immune system will know what to do. It's just about unleashing it from the constraints." Allison's and his colleagues' findings in mice experiments, published in* Science *in 1996, promisingly declared that "it is clear that CTLA-4 blockade enhances antitumor responses." Translation: This stuff works. And as Allison told Jerome Groopman in the* The New Yorker *in 2012, "I just wanted to be the advocate who is keeping it in everybody's face."*

Nils Lonberg recalls it similarly. Lonberg is currently a senior vice president of biologics discovery at Bristol-Myers Squibb, but he's been delving into the mysteries of the immune system his entire career. On a swampy late summer afternoon in 2014, he and I are sitting in a room at BMS's New York headquarters, where he tells a story that for him begins back in grad school.

"I'll go back to 1989," he says. "I was at Sloan Kettering. Jedd Wolchok was doing a summer internship in Alan Houghton's lab, the lab that Wolchok now runs. I was downstairs working on genetically engineering mice. I was talking to people who were working with a mouse monoclonal antibody. The problem they were having was that our human bodies recognize them as foreign proteins. So I asked whether it would be useful to have a mouse that could make human monoclonal antibodies—if I could genetically engineer a mouse that would have human immunoglobulin genes, rather than mouse immunoglobulin genes. And," he says modestly, "there was enthusiasm there."

Though Lonberg speaks of this process with all the easy confidence that I generally employ when I'm offering to make a tray of cupcakes for a bake sale, it's actually kind of a big deal to get animals to make human antibodies. It took Lonberg and his several associates years to get there. It was also an eminently hands-on process. Researchers had to isolate a specific part of the immune system code inside human DNA, inject it into mouse embryos, and then blow those embryos into mother mouse oviducts via a tube—a feat Lonberg repeated on tens of thousands of mice. "It is personal," he tells me. "You get in there, and someone actually has to do that." Lonberg and his team's results on the mouse that could make human antibodies, published in 1994, were groundbreaking.

"There are now," he says, "six approved antibodies that came from that mouse. There's a psoriasis drug. Another is an arthritis drug." And there's Yervoy.

The next step was getting the antibodies into patients. "Alan Korman talked to Jim Allison shortly before Jim's paper came out in 1996," he says. Korman is now the vice president of discovery research at Bristol-Myers Squibb, and was at the time, like Lonberg, at the pharmaceutical company Medarex. "He became immediately enthralled. Jim had had frustration getting other people interested in this, but Alan was very interested. Alan had made a mouse monoclonal antibody, and he wanted to manufacture it to take it into the clinic. I gave him some advice about manufacturing, but I said, 'You don't really want to put a mouse antibody into patients. You want to put a human antibody into patients. Let's make a human antibody.' "

Lonberg recalls an early meeting with James Allison. "He was really skeptical of all the promises he'd been made by the biotech industry, and his primary concern was that he was obsessed with getting this into patients as soon as possible. The first patient was treated with ipi in June of 2000. All the time to negotiate a three-way agreement between [Allison's lab in] Berkeley and [pharmaceutical companies] Nextar and Medarex, all the time to work on the drug, to manufacture it for the clinic, the regulatory filing, the toxicity studies—all that was compressed into less than two and a half years. We were so urgent." Nevertheless, in the more typical pace it generally takes for drugs to clear all their hurdles in the United States—though that's now beginning to change—it would take more than a decade of trials before the treatment that became ipilimumab would be approved by the FDA.

When I talk to people like Lonberg or Allison or Wolchok, I see real humans doing things like blowing embryos into mice in the name of the rather amazing cause of developing new treatments for cancer. That's why I really have to restrain myself when people go all conspiracy theory on me. I have to bite my tongue when a neighbor who overhears me talking with Jeff about my drug trial in the elevator one afternoon pipes up to say, "I don't believe in drugs. Any of 'em. The cancer doesn't kill people. It's the drugs." Or when on the playground one blustery afternoon, a fellow mom pityingly sighs at me as our daughters play and says, "It's terrible you're going through this. These doctors. They don't want to find a cure."

"I'm sorry, what?" I ask.

"The doctors," she continues, "the drug companies, they're all working together to keep people sick. They make more money treating cancer than they could to cure it. If they cure it, they're out of business. All this money

goes to research, so why isn't there a cure?" Tip: This is the opposite of what you should ever say to someone with cancer.

"Gee," I reply, "I've got to say it's a very convincing hoax. My doctors have spent their whole adult lives allegedly investigating treatments and the researchers working on drug trials have done the same. It's pretty impressive to think they're really just sitting around letting everybody die. Totally had me fooled."

"Well, no," she says hastily, "that's not what I meant."

"You haven't been there," I tell her, "and you don't know what you're talking about."

I would never claim that any industry that is profit driven doesn't very much look out for its own interests. A popular drug—a drug there's proven demand for—makes people money. That's why, whenever there's a big breakthrough in medicine announced in a prominent section of the news, there's always a smaller but still significant story farther down about how the pharmaceutical company's development will affect investors. And yes, I get that it's undeniably weird that a large corporation's financial success is often riding on the investment in the chance that people like me won't die, but there it is.

In 2009, Bristol-Myers Squibb purchased Medarex Inc., the small pharmaceutical company that it had been co-developing ipi with, for $2.4 billion. That's not a choice anybody makes emotionally. That's a choice heavily influenced by, as an analyst at Credit Suisse noted to Forbes *at the time, the promise of "future royalty streams." As researcher friend Steve says, "The way it works in real life is that we're capitalists. I have a fiduciary responsibility to the stockholders to not do anything stupid and risk their investments."*

That means hard realities, but it doesn't mean everyone involved in drug development is a ghoul. Shortly after Yervoy was approved in March 2011, one of the doctors at Memorial told me that a neighbor who works on Wall Street had confronted him in his apartment elevator one morning on the way to work. "You know," the neighbor had said, "the Street hates your drug."

"I didn't say anything," he had told me, "because what would be the point? But I thought, first of all, it's not my drug. Second of all, I don't work for the Street. I work for my patients."

There is a lot about the drug industry, about the insurance industry, and about the relationship that many of us as patients subsequently are forced to have with our wellness and illness that is radically screwed up. That is not the same as an elaborate plot. As Jedd Wolchok says, "All the things that you may think you know and understand about clinical trials, about pharma, about the health care system, about cancer—you can't know it until you're 360 degrees surrounded by it. You're definitely not going to know it by reading someone ranting and raving on the Internet."

CHAPTER 16

The Trial

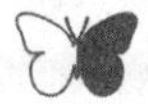

October 8, 2011

By the time we drive down to Philly on Saturday, I am feeling almost not awful. As the car glides over the George Washington Bridge, Jeff drives as I fiddle with the car radio until I land upon Captain and Tennille. He and I reflexively belt out "Love Will Keep Us Together" with such disquieting gusto the kids can only sit slack-jawed in the back at our display. "I will! I will! I will!" we sing-shout. I am thinking of nothing else in the whole wide world, and it's fantastic.

Deb's just started on her course of Abraxane, but when she emerges from the house, sliver thin and bandanna wearing, I don't feel the same scared butterflies I did in May. I just feel proud of how hard the two of us worked to get here, right now.

Tonight, our families laser tag. Debbie and Mike and Jeff and I suit up together, and before long we're obliterating our children with extreme prejudice. I pull the trigger so often and so fast that I'm more often than not shooting blanks, rushing back to recharge and relishing the thrill of faux annihilation. Of being, for a change, the killer.

Debbie, ever the beanpole, has lost even more weight since May. As we putter around the next morning before breakfast, I notice how her jeans sit low on her hip bones, and how, peeking out between the top of her belt and the bottom of her shirt, I can see a dark vertical scar.

"So that's it," I say, glancing at her abdomen, and she tugs down her shirt hurriedly, embarrassed. But then she seems to remember how superfluous modesty has become, and she pulls up her shirt, revealing her belly with all the finesse of a girl on spring break, going wild. She pats it proudly.

There is a long, straight line from her chest to her pubic bone, flanked by two deep parallel scars on either side. It looks like an upside-down cross.

My eyes follow the trail of marks down the front of her body, and then back up to meet her eyes.

"Plus, I'm losing my hair again," she says.

"Yeah, where's Ellen?" I ask. She's not on her old spot on the bookcase.

"Oh, I don't know what to do about her," Debbie says. "All my students have seen me with short hair already. I don't know if I can walk in with a pageboy. I guess I have to go back to Lovely You and get something in a pixie."

"It's all impressive," I say, lifting my shirt too. "Better than mine." I point to the little gashes on my left side, under my armpit, and under my breast. "And this," I say with a flourish as I swivel around to my right side, "is my tumor."

"That thing?" she asks incredulously. "It looks like a little bruise."

"Right?" I say. "It's hard to believe that it's actively trying to kill me."

After we're all dressed, we go out to breakfast at a local diner. I may have Stage 4 cancer, but with a treatment plan in place, I am beginning to *feel* better. The eight of us sit together laughing and talking over each other and ruthlessly grabbing food off each other's plates, and buttered raisin bread and I even rekindle our lifelong romance. But as Debbie's family and mine walk toward the cars to head back to our respective homes and the prospect of my Monday morning return to Sloan Kettering hits, suddenly so does the fear and the anger at the colossal number cancer has been doing on Debbie and me for the past year. The bandanna on Debbie's head, the way she's still in treatment. The relief of yesterday gives way to the inevitable fear and anger. And anxiety. Our families walk to the cars, and we promise to see each other again as soon as possible. I wonder if we will, though. See each other again, I mean. Cancer has a way of changing your relationship with the future and your plans for it. I watch Debbie get into her car as we all pile into our rental. I scoot the kids into the backseat, and then I climb into the passenger side. I don't even get the door closed before I burst into tears.

The tears are so sudden and excessive that Jeff and the kids are alarmed. "Are you okay?" Jeff says. "Do you need to wait here awhile?"

"Just go," I reply. "Drive. Please."

We cruise right behind Debbie for a few blocks, until we come to the intersection where we have to turn and she must keep going straight on. She pulls up right next to us on her left-hand side. There are tears and mascara sliding down my face, but when she honks her horn, I attempt a valiant smile and wave through the car window. Obviously, she can tell how hysterical I am right now; she's being polite as she gamely waves back. She'll later tell me that no, in fact she couldn't tell, because she was too busy crying herself. "I cried the whole way home," she'll say, a feat I find impossible to envision because I have never, in all the time I've known her, seen her even a tiny bit verklempt. "I thought for sure I'd never see you again." I tell her that I had thought that too.

As soon as we come home, down the rabbit hole I go. While my aggressive cancer cells continue to do their work in my body, I embark on a punishing back-and-forth regimen at Sloan Kettering. Urine tests. X-rays. EKGs. An insane number of blood tests that fill vial after vial for collection. I do it all while working and parenting and trying to hold together the rest of my life. And I don't for a minute take it for granted that both my job and my family are incredibly accommodating of my inconvenient, crummy health situation. I know not everyone gets that level of support.

There are also consultations with Dr. Wolchok and the trial team. I meet my no-nonsense trial nurse Karen and two of my team fellows: a whip-smart young doctor named Evelyn, and a young man with pearly teeth and good hair whom I will call Dr. Pete to his face and Dr. Handsome to my friends. I am not convinced he is yet mature enough to rent a car, let alone treat my melanoma.

"How old are you?" I ask him bluntly.

"I'm 30," he replies.

"That's a nice age," I say. "You know what happens in your 40s? You get divorced, you get cancer, and your parents die."

"I'll . . . keep that in mind," he replies politely.

In the blur of my days at Sloan Kettering, I even, at last, meet the chair of the immunology program, the famous Dr. James Allison. It is not a momentous event when I do. He just happens to be strolling by the front desk while I'm talking to Dr. Wolchok. "This is somebody you need to meet," Dr. Wolchok says, but he doesn't mean I should meet Allison. He means Allison should meet me. "This is one of our new candidates for the combo trial," he says, smiling toward me. It's extremely cordial, but I cannot help feeling that my dire diagnosis is there in the subtext.

I am not a particularly superstitious type, but knowing that the head of this medical team is an Allison provides me a comforting sense of symmetry. Exactly one year before my diagnosis, a dearly loved friend died suddenly and much too young. Her name was Allison. It feels right to have this new and very different Allison in my life. This Allison has white hair and small, neat glasses and a Texas accent. He's probably the smartest human being I will ever come face-to-face with—and when I meet him my first impression is that I like him because he looks like a troublemaker. "Pleased to meet you," he says in his honeyed southern drawl, and then he saunters off again. There's something about the guy that seems a little wild and dangerous and makes me feel safe. He's the feisty Mick to Dr. Wolchok's cool Keith.

Not everybody here has that effect. For another one of my appointments, Dr. Wolchok is out of town at a conference, so I am sent for the day to a different doctor. Dr. Fields is an elegant Dr. Oz type who exudes TV star confidence and comes with his own entourage.

"I've brought some of our residents here today to observe, if that's all right with you," he says, pointing to a group of five very young-looking strangers.

I nod my assent. I'm part of research already. It would be silly not to acknowledge that I'm here for the doctors to learn from.

Dr. Fields tells the residents, in dry terms, about the cancer in my lung and on my back, recounting the Case of the Metastatic Melanoma. Then, pointing at me, he tells the group, "Let's get a look at the tumor." Apparently I am the tumor. I obligingly lift up my seersucker. "Ah yes," he says with a nod as his posse flutters around me. "So we have a 2.5-by-1-centimeter unresectable tumor on the right chest wall." He touches it and it's sore.

"Dr. Partridge told me they can remove it if I want," I pipe up.

He looks genuinely startled, and I cannot tell if it's over this new development or the fact that the tumor is speaking.

"Oh, no," he says firmly. "You have to let us know what you're planning on doing, because we need that tumor for our study. It's your only visible site of disease, so that makes it a useful marker for us to measure our progress. If you remove it, you can't be in the trial. But," he adds condescendingly, "it's your decision."

There's no windup. No "Let's talk this over." Just an unpleasant person who seems not to give any damns that I am a human facing a serious disease. I'm not really here to meet your "needs," I think, but I say, "I thought I could do both the procedure on my back and still be in the trial, because of the cancer in my lung. Dr. Partridge never said it would disqualify me. She told me we could do an in-office procedure; she said it to me while she was working on getting me into this trial."

"No," he says again. "We need both the tumor on your lung and the one on your flank." Like I'm a horse.

I'll still have to decide whether I want the surgery, but I know for sure one thing I definitely don't want. I am not Tina the Talking Tumor, and I don't give a rat's ass about what Dr. Fields wants in his glorious quest for medical advancement. I'm happy to help the cause of science, but not to the exclusion of what's best for me first.

I have already come so far in the process, but they cannot make me do the trial. "Well, I'll think about what you've said," I tell him, "and I'll get back to Dr. Wolchok with my decisions."

He nods. "You can get dressed now," he says to the door as he walks toward it, his flock trailing behind him. I put on my clothes, and on my way out, I stop by the front desk with a message. "I won't be seeing Dr. Fields again," I say to Cal, the office manager. "I don't want to talk to him and I don't want him to touch me. So please make a note of it." I never see him again. A year later I will read a newspaper interview with him and decide that he sounds like a brilliant and dedicated researcher—and a total cocky douche.

For the grand finale of my pretrial testing, I do an MRI over at the main hospital. I am put into a tube, get injected with a solution that immediately makes me want to vomit, and have images of my brain taken while I spend the next half hour listening to a clanging din. Then they send me downstairs for my CT scan. I drink my jug of contrast dye, change into a robe, get hooked up to an IV, and wait in a crowded hallway with the other patients. I sit there next to a little girl who is whining to her mother. The girl cannot be older than four. She is as tiny and breakable looking as a baby bird. She is bald and shivering under a blanket. I glance over at her and her mother stoically fussing with her covers.

"I want to go home," she pouts. "You said we weren't going to be here this long. I'm cold I'm cold I'm cold!"

"I'm sorry," her mother says. "We'll be done soon."

Across from us, a hollow-cheeked, dark-haired young woman is lying down on a stretcher, staring blankly into the middle distance and breathing laboriously. She seems entirely unaware of the other woman, the one who looks like a healthy version of her, holding her hand. I suppose they're sisters. God, I hate this. I hate that we're here, on a cloudless October morning, with saline in our veins and contrast dye in our stomachs. But we're here to get better, I tell myself as the tears begin to sting my eyes yet again. We're here to heal. I have to allow for the possibility that this child and that young woman are going to be okay. For their sake, and the sake of the ones who love them.

When it's all over, no one tells me officially that I'm accepted into the trial. There is no congratulatory letter that arrives, preferably via an owl. There is no lottery winning–like ebullience in the message. They just call me in for another screening consultation and mention that the MRI was clear. "Nothing in your brain but your brain," the technician says.

I have aced the mysterious vetting process, proving myself sick enough yet fit enough, while also meeting other, more ephemeral qualifications. The first thing I had going for me was just a willingness to show up. Dr. Pete tells me later, "Lots of people hear the words 'clinical trial' and it freaks them out." I know, because I was one of them.

He continues, "It's about patients being interested, understanding what it is that they're participating in, and being motivated to follow the trial protocol. We need patients who will take the pills as prescribed or come to their appointments as scheduled. If a patient wants more flexibility in their care, that's more than reasonable, but maybe Phase 1 trials are not right for them." And when I ask him if age is a factor, he says not really. "You can be 40 years old and you have something that may make you not a good candidate, or be a patient who's 75 who's an excellent candidate, no problem. Functional age is just as important as a numeric one."

For the next step before I can start getting some drugs in my cancer-riddled body, I meet with a tiny, dark-eyed nurse who reminds me of Wednesday Addams in a lab coat. She hands me a 27-page document explaining my treatment plan and every possible side effect they've considered. Of course, because this drug combination is virtually untried on humans, there may be others that surprise us. "It's all pretty standard. This is just in case, you know, your head falls off or something, ha ha," she says, but I don't laugh. Among the "likely" side effects are fever, low or high blood pressure, sweating, rash, itchiness, shakes/chills, fatigue, decreased appetite, and diarrhea, which apparently is so very likely it's printed in bold. Other "less likely" effects include vomiting, dizziness, and shortness of breath. Under "rare but serious" possible side effects are autoimmune disorders, lung inflammation, acute kidney injury or failure, multiple organ failure, and meningitis. I am also warned I cannot take herbal supplements or do acupuncture or get a flu shot. Maybe my head will fall off or something.

I fill out all the forms, including the one that says, "You will be asked to take part in this study for life." I fill out the one that asks, "Are you the only person responsible for minor children and unable to care for them?" I am not the only person responsible for my children, and I can care for them just fine. Yet the implication of the question, the issue of potentially leaving one's offspring, hits me like a brick. I sign off on everything, asserting that I understand the risks, that I consent to have my blood and tissue studied, that I am entering into what in the very best possible case scenario is a very long relationship. As I leave, I am handed a printout of a schedule. It has me down for two full years of active treatment, and follow-up appointments with dates years into the future. I wonder how many of them I will live to keep. "You'll be with us forever," the nurse says with ominous cheerfulness. You can check out any time you like, but you can never leave.

It's becoming very real to me that this will not be easy, even though being in the first cohort means I am to receive the lowest dosage combination. I had wanted to be closely watched, and, by God, I will be scrutinized beyond my wildest dreams. The hope is that the dose is high enough to be effective but low enough to not have a battery of other consequences.

Here's another thought: Even if this bombs out and I'm dead in a few months, maybe my messed-up, diseased body can be of use to somebody else. Somebody who's getting a phone call today from a doctor who's telling her, "I'm sorry." I am a patient, but I really am a medical experiment too. I'm like one of Nils's little mice—as Dr. Fields's behavior rather tactlessly reminded me. But I like the idea of being helpful, even if I'll never really know exactly how. As Dr. Pete tells me later, as we sit in the afternoon sun in a conference room at Sloan Kettering, "We're doing so many studies now on the melanoma samples we've collected from patients, and looking at different mutations in them. That is a big part of the scientific literature." I am not Mary Elizabeth anymore; I'm not even Mary. I'm Trial Patient Number 1626. I'm your bitch now, science.

I'm still hopeful for a brighter fate than being just a lesson from an experiment, though. Just as Dr. Partridge once told me, it is indeed a terrific time in melanoma. Dr. Wolchok will later explain to me, "I spent the first decade of my career dealing with medicines that had a vanishingly small chance of helping someone—and when they did help, they didn't help for a long period of time. The world changed in 2010, because of ipilimumab and also because of the BRAF inhibitors [like vemurafenib]: two different approaches to treating melanoma, both of which were rapidly approved by the FDA because both were demonstrated to improve overall survival. This had never been shown before in medicine to treat metastatic melanoma. Melanoma is teaching us a lot about how all of the things we believe we know about cancer may be untrue." In the United States in 2011, roughly 70,000 new patients will be diagnosed with melanoma. More than 9,000 patients will die of it. That's one person every hour. I have been accepted into the first cohort of this Phase 1 trial. There will eventually be 53 people in my arm of the trial—but right now, there are fewer than a dozen enrolled. They will range in age from their early 20s into their 80s. Because I am considered relatively young and healthy, because I live where I do and have the cancer center I have, I now get the chance to be one of them. So suck on those odds, cancer.

CHAPTER 17

Hotel California

October 13, 2011

I'm in the waiting room in my FUCK CANCER shirt and magical butt-flattering Lululemon Groove pants, which is as close to being in my pajamas in public as I feel I can pull off. Today is the first day I'm finally getting these mysterious drugs I've been hearing so much about, and I want to be as comfortable as possible for it.

For the initial week, I will go to Sloan Kettering four out of five days so they can give me the treatment—an infusion of one drug, and then the other—and monitor me and take my vitals and my blood. If all goes well, I will then go back for monitoring, blood work, and/or treatment at least once a week, every week, from now until the springtime, so they can make sure I'm not losing weight or my liver is not staging a rebellion.

I'm not the only rookie here. Directly across from my chair is a dark-haired, blue-eyed young man who isn't even trying to conceal his secret identity. He's wearing a dark T-shirt with the numbers 007 on it. "Nice shirt," I say.

"You too," he replies. His is name is Frank. He's 24, and this is his third recurrence. He's already done chemo and interferon and the ipi alone, and nothing stuck. He's brought in his laptop today, and confides that he's told his office he's taking a work-from-home day because he's afraid of the career consequences if they find out he's sick. "I don't talk about it with the people at my job," he says. "I don't talk about it much with my friends either. They don't really get it." Everybody I know has an intimate relationship with cancer. I cannot imagine how lonely it must be for someone young like Frank. Fuck cancer, indeed, in so many ways.

For my first stop, I meet with Dr. Wolchok and Nurse Karen, and then go back to the treatment area and am introduced to my new team of nurses: Susan, a Bay Area native who's supposed to be preparing for retirement but says she loves the work too much to stop; Naomi, a divorced mother of two young children; and Christie, a fresh-faced recent nursing school grad from the suburbs who tells me, "It's the craziest day. I just ran into a guy I went to high school with. It's his first treatment day too." I'll bet it's crazier for Frank.

I am disheartened when I am told I cannot go out for lunch but perk up when they hand me a deli menu and tell me I can order anything on it. On the one hand, I have forfeited my emancipation today, cooped up in a chemo suite. On the other hand, my appetite has been coming back, and there's free soup. I can also have all the Shasta I want from the kitchen. It's a mite disingenuous, however, that they call my humble cell a "suite," like Kanye is going to show up with a bottle of Dom and invite me to hang out on a white leather couch. Yet for a location whose defining characteristic is the giant IV tower, it's all right. There's a reclining chair and a TV and a window lined with potted plants. I have a sliding door that I can close to tune out the noise from the nurses' station. I have brought my laptop and there's free Wi-Fi, so while all the other chumps who don't have cancer are stuck working today, I have *American Horror Story* on Hulu. It's quite a racket I have going on here.

There's lots of checking my vitals and peeing in cups before we can officially get the party started. Naomi comes in with a large tray of tubes. She puts a needle in my arm and takes blood, and then she keeps on taking. "I've never drawn this much out of one person at a single time," she says, and I feel like an overachiever. She will do two smaller though also damn impressive additional blood draws before the day ends for a grand total of 36 vials. USA! USA!

It's lunchtime before my drug cocktail comes back from the pharmacy and they even start the first infusion. I have a blood pressure cuff on my arm and an IV line in the other when Naomi rolls in with a bag that says "High Alert." She and Christie cross-check the name on my bracelet against the name on a form and recite the protocol number, and then at last I feel a rush of saline entering my body and a telltale metallic taste in my mouth, the opening act for the drugs themselves. It's cool, and startling, like an ice-cream headache in my veins. Get in there and do your thing, drugs, I think. My T cells are ready to greet you and to go on an internal killing spree.

The rest of the day involves a lot of mechanical beeping and getting tangled in a mess of cords while the blood pressure cuff periodically inflates. On this first day, I will be at Sloan Kettering for 12 hours, comfortable and scared and bored and very, very drained. Finally, as I leave in the evening, I pass by Frank's suite as he's wrapping up too. "See you next time, Mr. Bond," I say.

"Until we meet again, FC," he answers.

I will come back again and again this week, getting monitored and tested. Every time, the journey to and from Memorial will seem longer and more tiring. The side effects are kicking in quickly. This wouldn't be so bad, I had assumed. I have a strong constitution. I am in good shape. I will be one of those people who sails through this sort of thing. Then again, I tend to be wrong about a lot of things, especially when it comes to my cancer.

This morning I found myself absently scratching my forearm in the shower and discovered that overnight, a richly hued red rash had bloomed there. I was further surprised to note the places along my legs and arms where I'd clawed off my itchy flesh in my sleep. It's okay, I had thought, I can just dab it with the A+D ointment I've been stockpiling since the scalp surgery until I can get something stronger from the doctor. The funny taste in my mouth—a puckery, tannic sensation usually associated with strong tea or not great red wine—that's different. The breathlessness during my morning run—that strained, exerted feeling that doesn't usually start until several miles in or when I'm conquering a steep incline—that was new. It had been with me from almost the first moment my sneakered feet hit the pavement. It had dogged me like a hankie full of chloroform all during my train rides to and from 53rd and 3rd, as I sat listless and groggy on the A. Now, walking up Isham Street with Lucy and Bea this afternoon, I am suddenly all too aware of why they call this neighborhood Inwood Hill.

I haven't been this tired since my pregnancies. My pregnancies. So long ago now. Eight years since the last. I'm in my mid-40s now. I not only don't want any more babies, I know damn well my body most likely cannot make any more babies. But when, as I'd filled out all those release forms for the trial, my creepy Charles Addams cartoon nurse had asked, "You have your family, right? You're done having children?" and then added much more firmly, "You cannot get pregnant," something inside of me died a little. My "don't want to" became a "not allowed to." My most abstract, fuzzy-wuzzy concepts are now vividly real. I am never going to have another baby. I am going to die someday. Possibly soon. Really.

On the upside, I got through the first treatment and it didn't kill me. Only two more years to go—if I'm lucky. As a bonus, Dr. Wolchok called me yesterday to say he's had a conversation with Dr. Partridge, and that I am approved for the back tumor surgery if I should choose to do it. It won't affect my participation in the trial. I know she'd said it wouldn't change things much regarding my overall condition, so for now I'm going to wait and see. But I like feeling in the driver's seat of my own care, like knowing that Dr. Fields is not the boss of me.

The girls and I are now lurching past the playground when I spy Jolie with her kids. "You're not wearing your hat," she says. "I almost didn't recognize you." I haven't seen Jolie in months. It's been an eventful time.

"My hats were sacrificed in the big nit smothering of 2011," I say. "I haven't had any time to get out and get any new ones, because Sloan Kettering's been keeping me busy."

"I heard," she says gently. I always feel at ease around Jolie. Her experience as a nurse makes her unsqueamish around festering head wounds and hair vermin. Her empathy as a friend makes her priceless.

As our respective broods scamper off together, she asks, "So are you guys doing anything? As a family?"

I'm not sure if she's talking about the lice or the rediagnosis. I look at her blankly.

"I just know that when Andy and I were going through the D-I-V-O-R-C-E, it helped to have some extra emotional support."

"The girls are doing great," I reply. "They're so strong and so together." I think back to how Bea managed to be a comfort to me, even when she was bagging up her stuffed animals.

"I can tell," she replies, looking over at our children, frolicking carelessly. "But sometimes it's nice for kids to have somewhere they don't have to be great. Sometimes it's nice for everybody." She gives me a look that's both eminently kind and fiercely penetrating. "There's a place downtown," she continues. "A lot of my patients go there. Have you heard of Gilda's Club?"

"Maybe," I say. "It's for women with ovarian cancer, right?"

"Not just them," she answers. "Anybody affected by cancer. Patients. Families. It's helped a lot of patients I know."

"Thanks," I tell her. "I'll think about it." But as soon as we get home, I am Googling "Gilda's Club." They have support groups for people with cancer, for their children, and for their caregivers. I remember Deb's and my conversation last spring, about how hard cancer can be on the people who don't have it. Maybe it's just my childhood fondness for Gilda's *SNL* characters Lisa Loopner and Emily Litella calling out to me now, or just a trust that Jolie sees something in the girls and in us that we need—but I know immediately when I look into Gilda's that I want us there.

Lucy, meanwhile, peers over my shoulder suspiciously.

"Are you going to try to make me talk about my feelings?" she asks. "Because if that's what this is about, I refuse to do it."

"Me too!" Bea chimes in, like a character out of A. A. Milne.

"Take it easy," I tell them. "Try to keep an open mind. I just want to check it out. You know, it's right by the gelato place." A look passes between the girls, one of their creepy telepathic sister things.

"That means it's near the pizza place too, right?" Lucy prods.

"I suppose it is," I coolly reply. Oh, they're in.

"Would Daddy come too?" Bea asks.

"I think it would be very nice if he did," I say, even though I haven't even talked to him yet about putting the family in a support group. He walks past Gilda's red clubhouse door every day on the way to work. Now it's time to walk in.

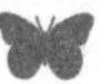

October 27, 2011

It's two weeks after my first treatment, and I'm at Memorial for monitoring again. Karen runs down a laundry list of side effects. "Itching?" Yes. "Rash?" Yes. "Diarrhea?" Ironically, not since I started the trial.

"Your bowels are otherwise okay? Because we need to know if there are any changes in your bowels."

"My bowels are amazing," I say. "If something happens, I promise you'll be the first to know."

Karen is all about my bowels. "We are obsessed with bowels here," she admits to me later. "I'll tell you, what ipi can do to someone's bowels is *unbelievable*. It's like a full-time job, literally, managing some people's bowels. As often as I can, I teach new people who are treating patients with something like ipi: bowels, bowels, bowels."

My bowels are currently holding their own just fine. There is something else going on, though. Something I've been scared to admit to myself, because what if I'm crazy, or just wrong? The discolored bump on my back. This morning I'd looked in the mirror after I stepped out of the shower and thought I saw something impossible. I called Jeff in and asked him, "Is it me or does my lump look different?"

He'd studied it intently. I could tell he was considering his words very carefully. "It's smaller," he said.

It's only been one treatment. We are hallucinating.

Yet when Dr. Wolchok asks, "Can we take a peek at your back?" his response is unhesitant and his delight is undisguised.

"Karen, look at this," he says. "Well, that is neat."

"Whoa," Karen assents. "Look how much it's gone down."

He peers at my back and then directly into my eyes. This must be what a ten-speed bike feels like on Christmas morning, because the expression on his face right now is not medical detachment. It's not unbridled elation either. It's the pure wonderment that one grants to a wish fulfilled.

"It's smaller," he says, just like Jeff did this morning. "Is this tender?" he asks, as he gently prods my flesh with his thumb.

"No," I say.

Three weeks ago, it was sore to the touch. There's no big whoop-de-do, no congratulatory handshaking. I just get off the table, gather up my purse and coat, and take my blown mind back to where I need to go next. This isn't all in my head. This is happening.

Three nights later I am at Fanelli's with Chez. Chez is a journalist and TV producer who lives in Miami. We became friends after he called me a humorless feminist on his blog, and I wrote him an email to call him a dismissive apologist for the patriarchy. Somehow we clicked. Chez has in his past three ex-wives and a benign but pinball-size brain tumor, and I currently have a fatal form of cancer, so whenever he comes to town we have plenty to bond over. It's still early in the evening when he asks how the trial is going.

"Not bad," I say. "I've got a crazy rash and I'm wiped out, but now I think I'm over the hump." I lean in to whisper what I'm still afraid to say out loud, afraid of jinxing it all. "I know it's nuts, but I think I may be improving. The tumor on my back, it's weird."

Chez, ever the newsman, demands evidence. "Let me see," he says.

It's been a while since I've lifted my top in a bar, but it turns out it's just like riding a bike. I reach my hand to the hem of my T-shirt and slide the back of it up to the place over my ribs where the mark is.

"I don't see anything," he says.

"It's a purple line," I tell him. "It looks like a bruise." I poke my finger to the place I know it is, though it's difficult to isolate precisely. Just a few days ago I'd have had no trouble locating it by its tender throb alone.

"Nope," he insists. "Believe me, honey, I'm looking. There's nothing there."

I turn my head back and meet his puzzled gaze. "Well, that," I tell him, "calls for another drink, don't you think?"

November 1, 2011

For our family's first night at Gilda's Club, we go for pizza and gelato beforehand, just as I'd promised the girls. They still don't seem that into the idea of a support group, but like their mother, they can be talked into almost anything if there's a melted cheese incentive somewhere in the deal.

Afterward, we stroll over to the cozy-looking building in the West Village, ring the bell, and are ushered inside. The four of us scan the lobby with a first-day-of-school nervousness. It's a small but inviting room, warmly lit and intimate. Two little boys are wrestling each other while their mother sprawls on the couch, casting heavy-lidded glances from underneath her ski cap in the direction of their shenanigans. The big one looks a year or so younger than Bea. I'd estimate his brother is just out of diapers.

A sunny, soft-spoken young woman with shiny, brown hair emerges from a doorway leading downstairs to the kids' club called Noogieland. "I'm Emily," she says, extending her hand first to me and then to Jeff before turning to the girls. "You must be our new Noogies. Come with me." She looks over at the boys. "You too, Zeke and Mo."

"Daddy and I have to go up to our groups now too," I tell the girls. "Have fun tonight."

Lucy gives me a hug, and as she does, she leans in toward my ear. "If they try to make us talk about our feelings, we're not coming back," she stage-whispers.

The woman on the couch looks amused. She hoists herself up wearily and heads toward the elevator with the grown-ups. "They'll be fine," she says, "if my boys don't wear them out."

"I'm Mary Elizabeth," I say, extending my hand. "Metastatic melanoma. It's my first night. This is Jeff. Caregiver, with a side of dead dad grief."

"Cassandra," she replies. "I have Stage 4 breast cancer."

"Sorry I just missed your special month," I reply, and the way she rolls her eyes tells me immediately I've found a comrade.

The elevator ascends, and Jeff and I part to enter our respective rooms. In mine, our serene-looking facilitator, Marlena, is already perusing the sign-in sheet and looking at her watch. Soon the other members of the group file in. The retired teacher. The songwriter. The dot-com entrepreneur. We are an odd assortment of humanity that would never have found ourselves in the same room if we didn't have this one thing in common. Yet within minutes of conversation, it's clear we have so much we share—the challenges of parenting, the demands of relationships, the struggles of ambition, and the balancing act of dealing with it all while facing our illnesses. By 8 p.m., I have a new family.

I feel an instant affinity for all of these people, but I like Cassandra first and best. I like the way she plants herself into her place on the couch in our meeting room with a New Yorker's territorial ruthlessness. I like that she is cranky and sardonic and unflinchingly tender when she speaks of her children.

Afterward, Jeff and I meet up in the hall. "How'd yours go?" I ask.

"It was . . . fine," he answers. "They're a good group. I feel like I can't say it to too many people outside that you've got Stage 4 cancer and *I'm* so tired. In there it was totally normal. But there's no way that confronting mortality for two hours isn't heavy."

Fortunately, the kids have been doing nothing of the kind. They are beaming when we pick them up downstairs, as Cassandra's boys run amok around them.

"Did they make you talk about your feelings?" I ask Lucy.

"No," she laughs. "We ate popcorn, and then we played with doggies." If you're going to put your kids in a support group because you have serious cancer, starting out on therapy dogs night is definitely the way to go.

"Jesus," I say. "Can I switch to your group?"

As we step outside, the relatively mild fall seems to have turned cruelly cold, and I shiver the whole way to the subway. When we get home, I crash into bed and am asleep before the children.

By Thursday, when I drag myself to treatment, I know something is up. "How are you doing?" Karen asks again as she runs through the list of side effects.

"Crappy, actually," I say. "I think I'm coming down with something, and it has nothing to do with my bowels. It feels like the flu."

I have my blood pressure checked, and it's my usual low number. My temperature is normal too. I have two dozen vials of blood drawn. While I wait for my cocktail of drugs to come up from the pharmacy, I go into the closet where they also store the greatest machine in all of Sloan Kettering, the blanket warmer—and grab myself a throw that feels fresh from the dryer. I return to my chemo suite and curl up with the first season of *Sherlock* on my laptop.

When Susan comes in to check on me, I say, "Listen, I'm not feeling too great. While I'm waiting, do you think I could go downstairs to the Duane Reade and get some Tylenol?" The fact that I am in a world-class medical facility, where they probably have access to Tylenol, doesn't enter my mind.

"Sorry," she says. "You can't have anything that would interfere with the treatment." She takes my temperature again and it's still normal. An hour later she and I repeat this scene almost verbatim. But by the time my first bag of drugs is wheeled in a short time later, I am shivering uncontrollably. And this time, when Susan takes my temperature, it's 103.

"Can I get a Tylenol now?" I ask grumpily.

"We need to send you to x-ray first," she says, "to make sure there's no infection." So I go to another floor and get some x-rays to rule out pneumonia, come back, and at last a young resident comes by bearing a tiny cup and two small, white, fever-reducing pills. "We can't do treatment today," he explains. "We have to wait to see how you're reacting." He looks over at my useless IV tower and the bag of ipi inside it, and the Tylenol in my hand. "Well, I'd guess this has been about a $25,000 day." Sorry about the high price tag, medical research.

I spend the next few days utterly miserable with fever and chills—and not a little terrified that my painstakingly documented experience at Sloan Kettering will raise enough concerns to get me kicked out of the trial. Fortunately, the crisis passes and nobody benches me. And although there's no way of saying definitively whether it was just one of the promised side effects of the treatment, my immune system going into overdrive, or an unusually wicked case of the flu, all I know is that as wretched as I feel, I'm not scared that this is a manifestation of my disease. I'm now hopeful that it's a sign of my improvement.

When I go back to Memorial the following week, I have a scheduled check-in with Dr. Partridge. "I've been hearing a lot about what's been going on with you," she says. "So let's take a look."

She runs her hand over the place on my ribs where, two months ago, there was a welt. "Look how that's gone down," she says, obviously impressed. "That Dr. Wolchok is going to put me out of business. Fortunately, I do a beautiful hernia operation."

December 9, 2011

We've never been a family big on Santa. In fact, Lucy's long held an active distrust of him, an aversion she's made plain since she told us, as a strangers-averse toddler, she did not want him to come to our apartment. Now she's almost 12 and mostly past the reindeer-on-the-roof phase of life anyway. But when Bea sat down recently at the dinner table to compose her Christmas list, Lucy had sat down next to her and written one too. When I'd asked to read it, she'd refused, saying that it was for Santa's eyes only—and that she wanted to see him. "Maybe I just want to tell him he sits on a throne of lies," she'd added, covering all her bases, belief and skepticism and *Elf* references–wise.

We'd trekked downtown to Herald Square, and it was everything *Miracle on 34th Street* and "SantaLand Diaries" had ever made me believe it would be—unbridled mayhem but also oddly sweet. We'd waited a long time as we snaked through an ersatz winter wonderland, until an adult dressed as an elf ushered us into a private area for a brief audience with Kris Kringle. The girls whispered wishes, and then the three of us sat together with him, smiling and laughing, for a photograph. We had Christmas and Santa, and going to Macy's with Mama. And though neither girl will ever tell me what they murmured into Santa's ear, I have a few ideas. I know what I'm wishing for this year myself.

Now, at the winter party in the homey backroom of our Gilda's clubhouse, the girls play with Cassandra's boys and their friend Donna, whose mother has Stage 4 colon cancer. The grown-ups sit together eating carrot sticks and cookies. I chat up Jeff's friend June from the caregiver group, and her wife, Evie, who has inoperable lung cancer. Across the room, Jeff chitchats with my musician friend Hugo and his stunning new girlfriend. Cassandra, meanwhile, holds court in the lobby, with the queenly air of someone who believes if you're worthy of an audience, you'll come to her. "Where have you been?" she asks when I flop next to her for a few minutes of snark and gossip. "I've been so bored."

"I was talking to Hugo," I say, "about the benefit concert he's putting together. How are you? How did the Neulasta shot go this week?"

"It was like," she says, as her eyes turn toward the snowflake decorations hanging from the ceiling as if they contain adjectives, "it was like I was on fire. Or like I was made of glass. And I was shattering."

"Yow," I reply. Sometimes, when I consider what people can live with and keep going, it shocks me. It's like after I had a baby, and realized that the world is full of exhausted women with lacerated perinea and clogged milk ducts who are managing to successfully keep small, helpless human beings alive. Now I know it's also full of people who go to the doctor and have shattering experiences and then show up with their kids for parties. Unbelievable.

"How are you feeling now?" I ask.

Cassandra is not one to mince words. "The truth is that I feel angry," she replies. "I'm angry at everybody who isn't sick. I'm angry that they get to live their lives and make plans and I'm too tired to play with my kids." She doesn't look good tonight, in her knit hat and sweatpants falling loosely over her thin frame. She reaches into her bag, pulls out her cell phone, and brings up a photograph of a chubby blond woman, smiling and holding a fat baby. I've never seen this woman. But I know exactly who she is. "That was two years ago," she says. "Back then, I wouldn't have gone near a thing like this." In another life, this all would have been way too lame for her. "And how are you?"

"Oh you know," I say, lightly. "Work. Treatment. Family. Holidays. Still just trying to be Wonder Woman."

She laughs, right in my face, at me. "Well, cut the shit," she says. "Wonder Woman didn't have cancer." She makes an excellent point. I never imagined that having it all would include having cancer.

At some point there's a raffle, and Lucy wins a lovely chemo scarf. Then Lily, the club's president, comes in to introduce three impossibly fresh-looking Julliard students. "We're going to play some songs for you," says a tiny Asian girl clutching a violin, right before she launches into "Amazing Grace."

God, what a cliché. I have never liked that song, not even as a devout, churchgoing child. It always seemed so flat and dirgelike, so wildly overused. Yet when I look around this room, on this night, at all these faces, it doesn't sound tired at all. For the first time in my life, I feel like I'm actually listening to the song—its first two words in particular. Amazing grace. Not soft and friendly, Hallmark card grace. Amazing grace. Like, blow your mind, rock your world, bring you to your knees grace. A Christmas ago, Dad was singing this song in church. A year from now, several of these people won't be here for the next holiday party, and that will forever change the lives of so many of the other people in this room. The spouses and the children and the friends and girlfriends and parents. Yet here we are tonight, a community united in friendship and devotion by the worst thing that ever happened to us. I sit back in my director's chair with the name of another member on the back, clutching a paper plate of Carr's crackers and bright orange cheese, rapt with amazement. And grace.

CHAPTER 18

The Valedictorian

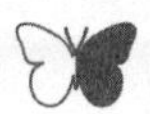

January 10, 2012

It's two weeks after Christmas, just a few days into the new year. The new year I have lived to see. It's the night I've won the cancer lottery. The night I will forever more hope to mark as my "Cancer free since . . ." date. My new birthday. Because I had my scans this morning, and I just got off the phone with Dr. Wolchok.

There's never an optimum location for bad news, but I could not possibly receive good news in a better place than right here at Gilda's Club, immediately before going in to my support group.

Our session tonight was surreal, in the nicest way. Everybody's got their own stuff going on, and some of it's really serious. Cassandra looks so tired lately. Ned has his big surgery next week. Yet my friends had all congratulated me, cried happy tears with me, when I told them that Dr. Wolchok had just informed me that my tumors are gone.

Downstairs, Noogieland is decorated with balloons and crepe paper. Tomorrow is the girls' birthday. As a preschooler, Lucy bragged to her friends about her baby sister before I was even pregnant. Her conviction was so convincing, like a Fox News reporter in heavy spin mode, that this other member of the family somehow seemed inevitable. Beatrice arrived on the morning Lucy turned four, an event they both describe as the best birthday present each ever got. When Lucy came to visit the hospital that afternoon, she regarded her new sister like she was a loved one who'd finally come home after a long time away. "There you are," she'd murmured, as she climbed into the bed with us. Bea snuggled right into her. They just fit.

Tonight, Emily and the other Noogies have thrown the girls a birthday party. Everybody is smiling and wiping cake crumbs off their mouths when Jeff and I walk in the room, ready to deliver the message from Dr. Wolchok.

I have learned not to say things to the girls like, "I have to talk to you," because it freaks them out. They are traumatized by the past year and a half of consistently horrible stuff. I will instead smile and say, "Mama just got some good news."

That was the idea, anyway. Unfortunately, as soon as I see my children, as soon as it sinks in that I get to keep being their mom a little longer, I promptly burst into overwhelmed, grateful tears.

"Oh my God, what's wrong?" asks Lucy.

"Mommy, what happened?" says Bea. "Is it bad news? Did someone die?"

I mutely gesture at Jeff, trying to indicate to tell them that it's all okay. "Nonononono," I burble, which doesn't help. Finally, I manage to get it out. "I'm cancer free. My scans were clear."

The kids look at their father, puzzled that Mom is basically behaving exactly like she does when she gets terrible news. They hug me tentatively as I just cry and cry like an idiot.

In my photo from that evening, the girls are sitting with their arms slung around each other, smiling. Their friend Donna is next to Bea, looking demure, and Zeke is on Lucy's side, making a goofy face. In just a few weeks, both Donna's and Zeke's mothers will be gone.

Two days later, I am back at MSKCC for treatment. Twelve weeks into my trial, and I'm a pro at this by now—I've got my yoga pants and extra-warm cashmere sweater on to keep me cozy, my laptop for watching escapist TV shows on Netflix, and a SmartWater in one hand and a fresh Jamba Juice in the other to fortify me for all the blood they're about to take out. It makes me think of the last time I had lunch with my friend Bruce. He had talked about how he's been doing since his company went under and his parents died, and he'd said, "I used to feel like I was waiting for my life to get back to normal. Now I see, this is my life now. So this is my normal." This is mine.

First, though, I have to get my vitals checked and consult with Dr. Wolchok, Karen, and the medical team. As I walk toward the examination room, I can feel the penetrating gazes of a row of interns and administrators. They're not even trying to be cool about it. I feel like I should be waving from a float while they toss rose petals at me. I knew they would be excited about my results, but it's not often you see such a celebratory mood on the cancer treatment floor. By the time I get to the exam room, I'm surprised that there isn't a sash and tiara waiting for me. A few minutes later, Dr. Wolchok walks through the door, looking considerably pleased.

I am, however, still in a state of cautious optimism. In cancer, we don't like to use words like "cured." We instead grudgingly bear the weight of other ones. Words like "recurrence rate" and "five years out." The memory of my kids pummeling me with kisses and declaring, "You're cancer free!" after my first surgery is a little too fresh. So when Dr. Wolchok says, "You present no evidence of disease" less than five months after being diagnosed at Stage 4 and just three months into treatment, I'm not entirely sure what to make of it.

"Tell me more about what the scans mean," I implore him. "You say the tumors are gone, but could there still be cancer in my bloodstream?"

He gives a "meh" face. "The idea with immunotherapy is that your system goes after the places there's disease," he explains. "If we're not seeing the cancer where we know it's been, we can assume it's not showing up anyplace else. We still don't have long-term data, but what we believe is that this treatment activates your immune system to keep defending itself in the future. It's not rocket science."

"Yeah," I say, "but it does seem to be curing cancer, and that's not too shabby."

The immune system learns, and it remembers. That's why I only got chicken pox once. The experience taught my body—the one I've lately been so angry at for turning on me so viciously—how to keep from getting it again. Now it's doing the same with cancer, kicking ass and taking names anywhere it suspects trouble. That's what this type of treatment does. The implications—not just for my cancer but other cancers—are almost limitless. Or, as my nurse Karen likes to put it, "It's the immune system, stupid."

Yet the urgent question remains: Why does this type of therapy work for some of us and not others? If any of the other handful of us doing this trial at MSKCC are anything like me, they've been dealing with scarred veins, side effects—and plenty of nagging uncertainty. Science is moving at a breathtaking clip, but when you've got a cancer that tends to kill within a year, it simply may not be fast enough for everybody.

"We had two other patients who had scans this week," Dr. Wolchok continues. "Both of their tumors have shrunk significantly. But you're at 100 percent, so for now that makes you our valedictorian."

"I'm just here to win," I say.

He nods. "Well, congratulations," he says. "Because, believe me, when a person with Stage 4 cancer has a complete response, that gets our attention." Oh, mine too.

I figure today I can hear it. Today, I need to. "So, exactly how bad is Stage 4?" I ask Dr. Wolchok. "Because Dr. Partridge says it's not what it used to be."

For once, Dr. Wolchok looks at a loss for words. "Ah, well," he stammers. "People don't usually ask me in those terms. They generally want to hear how bad it *isn't.*"

"Yes, but I'm your medical miracle, and I want to know."

He nods. "Melanoma cells are pretty tough. Think about it—they're what give you your skin color. They're designed to change and adapt and move around. That's why they're so resistant to conventional treatment. With other cancers, they often follow a predictable path. You rarely hear about cancer spreading into the small intestine or a tumor in the heart. With melanoma, you do." He pauses, searching for a phrase that will convey the seriousness of my case without making me launch into a full-blown panic attack. "You had a growth in your lung and an aggressive subcutaneous tumor, so we knew this thing wasn't fooling around. Your original tumor in your lung was growing. And," he adds, "there was the new one on your back."

I ask, "Was the tumor on my back the game changer? Did it mean the cancer was progressing much more quickly?"

"Not necessarily," he replies, cautiously. "Of course, any new tumor, regardless of where it is, compels you to do something. But I've never been a fan of counting the number of tumors that a person has, because the treatment that I'm usually offering people is one that affects the whole body. I try to reel people in from the numbers because the numbers can be very overwhelming." He's a diplomatic man. Though he will never say it to me directly, he'll later mention in an interview, "The textbooks would say that a patient with metastatic melanoma lives, on average, a bit more than a year."

"So what do I tell people now?" I ask him. "How do I describe where I am in this?"

"You can tell people," he says, "that you had a complete response." In cancer, a complete response means you have no detectable signs of disease. "You can tell them," Dr. Wolchok continues, "that you had Stage 4 cancer." Past tense. My official report from the CT scan, meanwhile, refers to my tumors as "resolved." I love the icy cool of that. It's a very mafia word, or maybe a Cold War spy one. Those cells that betrayed your body, Ms. W? They won't be bothering you any more. They've been "resolved." Which, in addition to being one of the best things that ever happened to me, is also a pretty damn fantastic—and not terribly common—thing to happen in the first cohort of a Phase 1 trial for cancer research. To a team of researchers and to Bristol-Myers Squibb, I am no longer the patient with Stage 4 cancer. I am the patient with solid results. I'm like Harry Potter, the boy who lived. I am the woman who did.

I am not the only one this is happening to. I just don't know the details yet. I don't know about the people from the original ipi trial who now, years after they completed it, are still thriving. I don't know about other patients like the one Dr. Wolchok later tells me about.

"This other gentleman—who doesn't even come back to see us anymore because he's out living his life—had a subcutaneous tumor he would point out to us every time he came in that kept getting smaller and smaller," he says. "Around the time of the fourth treatment, I said to Dr. Partridge, 'This guy is getting better, can you take this thing off his back? Because I can still feel it. It's a lot smaller, but I'm dying to know what's going on in there.' I remember there was a jaded surgery fellow working with her that day, and I ran up and asked, 'What did it look like? Was it all white cells?' He said, 'No, it was all black. It was just melanoma.' I walked away all dejected. Then I waited for the pathology report. It's still hanging on the corkboard above my desk. A 'histological picture of therapeutic success'—that was what the pathologist wrote to me. There was no melanoma left. There was just the pigment-laden debris. That was the beginning." He adds, "We also had people in your dose cohort who didn't do well. So it wasn't as if we had this expectation that you were going to do great too. But," and at this point he gives an eminently relieved shrug, "I could believe it."

That means that right now, there is the possibility that the middle-aged woman in Treatment Suite 26, the one whose elderly father sits by her side as they watch *Dr. Phil* together, is getting better. That the student in Suite 21, who endured a hellish year on interferon before he came here, is. That Frank, wearing his 007 T-shirt and talking to his old high school friend turned nurse in Suite 22, is too. That a whole lot more of us have the possibility that the fluid coursing into our veins is more powerful than the cells multiplying in our bodies.

This bleak winter morning is a quietly auspicious one. At a future CT scan, an oncology nurse elsewhere in Memorial Sloan Kettering will be chatting with me while taking my blood pressure and say, "You must be the one I've been hearing about." Months from now my friend Steve will tell me about being at a cancer event and hearing the buzz about, as he describes, it "some blogger lady with No Evidence of Disease." And Nils Lonberg will later describe to me seeing Dr. Wolchok at a conference in Washington, D.C., soon after and having him excitedly tell him about a woman in the trial he'd seen that week. As he recalls it, "Jedd was just hopping up and down. He came running over and said, 'We've got a complete response.' We were in tears." He will smile at the memory. "I bet that was you."

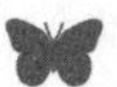

"So, do you want to see your scans?" Dr. Wolchok asks.

"Oh hell yes," I reply.

He sidles over to a monitor in the corner of the exam room and brings up an image. It's dated October 6, 2011. "This is your lung," he says. "See that there? That blob? That's the tumor." I peer at the screen. Well, hello, cancer.

He brings up another image right next to it. "This is it now." It looks just like the other one, but with one significant difference. No blob. He then does the same for the pictures of my back. "Here's the cancer," he says. There's a green arrow pointing to it, a flag that some radiologist added three months ago, a signpost of malignancy in my soft tissue. "And this," he says, double-clicking on a different picture, "is you now. Nothing." It's the most beautiful absence in the world.

I flash back to when I was pregnant with my daughters, gazing at sonogram images with my obstetrician. Here are your insides, I think. Here is your baby. Here is your cancer. Here is your life, changing dramatically just beneath the surface.

"Gosh," I say. "That's astonishing."

"Yeah," he says with a grin. "It's a lot more fun when it works." I look at the monitor. Yeah, it's just about the best fun ever.

February 2012

Goddamn it, I cannot do this. I just wanted a nice time out with my kid to see my hero, to show her the person whose songs I'm always poorly singing along with in the kitchen while I'm making dinner. I wanted to be non–cancer treatment mom for just a night.

We were going to see Debbie Harry. Of all the rock-and-roll heroes I've had in my life, she's my number one. Tough yet glamorous. New-wave goddess. Disco queen. Rap innovator. My Jersey homegirl. And tonight, she's doing a benefit show for Lucy's public school, performing with the school band. Living in New York City is a crapshoot, but the cancer hospitals are pretty sweet, and sometimes Debbie Harry steps in to sing for your kids. So there's that.

This afternoon I had picked up Bea from school uptown, and Jeff had picked up Lucy from school downtown. The plan had been that we'd meet up at the venue and do the switcheroo—I'd hand Bea off to Jeff, and then Lucy and I would go to the show together. But now, on the subway to 42nd Street, I know something is wrong. I am moving forward, but I am somehow watching Times Square slip farther and farther away from me, like I'm being pulled backward through a tunnel. Everything is getting smaller and more claustrophobic at the same time. By the time I get to the venue, I feel like I can barely stand up. It's the treatment. A fairly minor side effect, this occasional and sudden clobbered feeling, but it's still one to be reckoned with when it hits.

Jeff and Lucy wave when they see us approach, and then I see their expressions wince in unison as they look at me. They can recognize it now. I hate seeing that look on them, that troubled anxiety. I hate being this weak, out-of-control person who's okay one minute and then a mess the next. I hate that I have to work so hard to hold it together, and sometimes I still cannot hold it together anyway. There was that time before *The Muppet Movie* that I'd almost fainted on the A train. That time at the library with Bea, when the security guard had to help me down the stairs. The school party, when I'd had to leave abruptly because I was so short of breath. This is what winning at cancer looks like. And as I collapse into a taxi and take Bea all the way back home, I think that sometimes it pisses me off.

A few nights later, I am walking down Carmine Street on a Tuesday evening to meet up with Jeff and the girls at Noodle Bar before Gilda's Club. I have another treatment coming this week, and I am almost looking forward to it. That's how much I appreciate a day to do little more than sit in a reclining chair—and also how strangely attached I have become to the chocolate pudding I get with my lunch there. The kids, meanwhile, have been spending winter school break week at Gilda's Club's Camp Sparkle, a free day camp for the Noogies. I understand there may have been a trip to the wax museum today.

I'm almost at the restaurant when the phone rings. It's Emily, the facilitator from the children's group. "I don't know if you heard," she says, "but Cassandra died this weekend."

Cassandra had not been back at group since the night I got my big news, but I never thought she was gone for good. I thought she was tired, or bored. I thought she'd be back. I didn't even think it; I assumed it without concern or question, even when the increasing frailty was obvious. Because although it is one thing for grandfathers who are pushing 80 to die of cancer, I still don't want to believe that mothers of young children die of it too. I still don't want to believe it can happen to my friends. I don't want to believe that the woman who held my hand that night last month, who looked at me with such love and light and generosity in her eyes, was dying then. That I will never ever see those green eyes or hear that sarcastic honk of a laugh again.

"It happened quickly," she says. "Hugo said he saw her at chemo last week. But then she had to go into the hospital Friday, and she died Sunday. We're going to talk about it at Noogieland tonight. I wanted to tell you ahead of time so you can prepare Lucy and Bea. I know how much they love Zeke and Mo."

"We all do," I say.

I am sobbing when I walk into the restaurant. I park myself on a stool next to the family, in front of a bowl of noodle soup already waiting for me. I can barely croak out the words. "Cass died," I say. "Stupid cancer. Stupid stupid stupid."

Jeff and the girls instinctively dismount from their stools to wrap their arms around me. They barely knew Cassandra, so they don't cry. They're pained not at the loss of her but at my grief over it. I spoon noodles into my mouth, not because I'm hungry but because there is a bowl of soup in front of me so I'm supposed to eat it, and I honestly don't know anything else in the world at this moment. "Dammit," I mutter. "Goddamnit," I say, as large, salty tears drip into the bowl.

How is it possible to be so gutted by the loss of someone I knew such a short time? Yet when I think of Cassandra, I think of a phrase I heard long ago—a friend of the road. It's the companion you make in your journeys, the person you cling to in strange terrain, when the traveler next to you is your one constant. Your fellow adventurer. Jill and Debbie were my friends of the road a long time ago, when we met back in college. Laura was my friend of the road. I met her on an airplane ride to Prague. Becky was my friend of the road. I met her in a childbirth class. Cassandra was my friend of the road in cancer. She made this strange and harsh landscape better. Now my friend is gone, and the road seems longer and lonelier.

When I walk into the meeting room for group, I can tell my other friends don't know yet. I got the call ahead of time so I could tell the kids, could explain to them why their buddies Zeke and Mo aren't down in Noogieland tonight. The regulars have all filed in, and I take my usual place on the couch. Marlena will most likely make the announcement before we start. Then a new woman walks in. She is roughly my age, whippet thin and sporting a G.I. Jane haircut that immediately telegraphs: recently ended chemo. I stifle a gasp as she parks in Cassandra's place. Hugo and Isabel shift uncomfortably, anticipating Cassandra's inevitable wrath should she walk in and find her space occupied. But she's not coming. She is never coming again. I just don't want anyone else in her seat yet. I reach out my hand to the woman and introduce myself. I wonder if the rest of the group can tell I've been crying.

"I'm Jessica," she says. "I'm just coming back from ovarian cancer." She lives in Boerum Hill, in Brooklyn. She was diagnosed last May at Stage 3c. She finished chemo in November and recently started on Avastin, and now she's coming here because, she tells me, "I have my biological maintenance, and now this is my psychosocial maintenance. My daughter, Mina, is starting Noogieland tonight too."

I know what Cassandra would tell her, but she's not here, so it's up to me now. "She'll love it," I say. "If my kids don't wear her out."

Then the clock sweeps past the number six and our group time officially begins, and Marlena says she has something to tell us before we start. These little moments are so unreal, I think, the ones right before the bomb goes off. And then tissues are reached for. A sheet containing information about the memorial is passed around. Jessica looks bewildered and slightly horrified. This is what you get when you join a cancer club. Sometimes, shit gets real right away.

Afterward, a shell-shocked–looking Jessica and her bubbly seven-year-old daughter, Mina, walk to the subway with Jeff and the girls and me. As the girls run ahead down the street, I ask her, "Are you okay? That was a rough one to have as an intro meeting."

"I was a little rattled by *that*," she admits. "Frankly, tonight my primary concern was my daughter going into Noogieland and what it'd be like for her. When she heard about Gilda's, she said, 'You mean there are other kids whose parents have cancer? This is like the first day of school! Maybe I'll find a new best friend!' But yeah, when I saw people crying I thought, Does this happen every week?"

"It doesn't, I promise," I say, "but it does happen. I had someone in my group die in the first month. Jeff, I think you had a death the first night, didn't you? I don't know what I expected. I guess I thought,

I'm going to go someplace I can talk about my feelings, and then I learned that yes, I will, but guess what? We *all* have cancer."

"The good thing is that there's safety in numbers," she says. "But the horror is that not everyone is going to make it, and we're going to have to live through that." That's what we do when we outlive our friends. We will cry and we will feel relieved and we will feel guilty too. And that's how we'll get through it.

CHAPTER 19

Side Effects

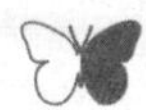

March 2012

The city is turning green early this year—winter had been so warm and mild, so damn near snowless—it couldn't resist bursting into color well before the official first day of spring. I lived to see the cherry blossoms after all. Cassandra's boys have now left the children's group. On their last night, the kids and Emily threw a going-away party for them. There was cake, and the kids made cards and sang songs and played games. It was so sweet and warm and joyful that every time I think about that going-away party—which is almost daily—I feel like my heart's being smashed to pieces. The boys are off somewhere else now, playing soccer and greeting the spring. Their first spring without their mother.

I'm here today at Memorial for another set of scans. They call my name and I head back to the women's waiting area to change. I surrender my clothes and walk past tiny examination rooms filled with snugly wrapped sick people. "Would you like a warm blanket?" the nurse says, proffering it, along with a stress ball, as she gestures to my chair. Don't mind if I do!

I settle in as she tries to jab a long needle into a vein in my right arm. "There's nothing there," she says, puzzled. Her face is furrowed with concern. "Can you squeeze the ball again, my love?"

I have known her about a minute, but, okay, I'll be her love. I take a quick glance at her name tag: Marie. I'll try to make my broken veins behave for you, Marie, but they were uncooperative, stingy little guys even before the cancer. The few IVs and blood draws I had in my old life were almost always punctuated by frustrated mutterings from the phlebotomist du jour. I swear to God, if I ever decide to become a junkie, I am totally sticking to smoking my heroin.

Now, however, my veins have achieved a whole new level of reluctance. Because of the trial, I have to come in every week for either monitoring or treatment. The nurses take alarming amounts of blood—dozens of vials at a time. I've been jabbed in a variety of exciting locations about my person. The crooks of both elbows. The middle of my forearms. The backs of my hands. Once, for a particularly memorable test of lung function, the artery in my wrist. My veins have been tapped and sapped on a more consistent, unrelenting basis than a keg at the end of Greek Week, and they are becoming hardened and blown out. Sometimes, I imagine Dracula stealing into my bedroom on a moonless night, slowly lowering his mouth onto my neck, and quickly pulling away with a disgusted "This is BULLSHIT."

Marie reties the piece of tubing around my left bicep this time, and I give the stress ball firm rhythmic squeezes as she firmly smacks the crook of my elbow, searching for a point of entry. Beads of sweat are forming on Marie's forehead now. She pushes the needle in and begins rooting around under the skin. I gasp in surprise at the sharp, clean pain as a tear spontaneously slides down my face. Marie looks horrified.

"I've been doing this for 25 years," she says, "and you're a tough one, my love. I'm so sorry, but I have to stop." She pitches unsteadily forward toward the sink as she adds, "I'm having a hot flash." She places a paper towel under a stream of water, and dabs at her neck and forehead. Apparently, I've just given my nurse menopause. "Would you like one too?" she offers, but I decline. She composes herself and asks, "Do you mind if we try it in your hand?" I look away as I feel the needle go in. I always thought "You can't get blood from a stone" was a figure of speech. I am a stone.

Marie leads me now to the CT scan tube as she shrouds my warm blanket around me like I'm the James Brown of cancer, delivering a bravura performance. I lie on the table. "Take a deep breath," an unseen voice commands. Seven seconds later it directs, "Let it out." Easy for her to say. After a few more times like this, the technician comes in and adjusts my IV. A metallic rush of saline floods my mouth and an icy charge shoots straight up through the vein in my arm. Then there it is. The warm, pissed-in-my-pants feeling strikes below. It happens every time, and every time I am positive I really have wet myself. It is the most mortifying conceivable possibility since I pooped a little on the bed somewhere in the throes of my first childbirth.

"You're done," the technician says. "Swing your legs around to the left and we'll help you off."

There's no puddle on the table. There never is. I still have a year and a half of treatment to go.

Afterward, trembling with chills, I go around the corner to cup my hands around an oversize bowl of ramen, and absently poke the yolk of the egg that floats on top. My dessert is a sweet jewel of *mochi* ice cream. I am strangely touched by it, feel oddly nurtured, as if the weird dollop of whipped cream on a lettuce leaf was meant as comfort just for me, an offering from my surrogate Japanese mother. I feel fortified and in control. An hour later I am walking back toward the subway when Dr. Wolchok calls to say I'm still clear. I am six months cancer free. And when you're on a virtually untested treatment protocol, it's still quite a novelty.

In some ways, I did get the good kind of cancer after all. I realize it when I am talking to James Allison on a summer day, right near the anniversary of my diagnosis, about why melanoma has been such a source of interest to researchers. I'd assumed it was because, as Nils Lonberg puts it, "There were no effective treatments for melanoma, so the immunotherapists were allowed to play in that little area. They weren't crowded out by the nonimmunotherapists, because there was just nothing there. We were given the playground that nobody else wanted to play in. We were dismissed. You would not believe it. It was terrible. At conferences we had the tiniest rooms." But Dr. Allison offers me another reason. "You work with melanoma because it's accessible. It's a bad disease," he says. "It has many mutations. People want to deal with it because it's so bad. It's rapidly fatal."

It's a vicious, unpredictable, and often swift-moving disease, and that makes it challenging to treat. It historically responds better to immune system–based treatments than other cancers have. And also, though Allison doesn't come out and say it, if a treatment for it isn't working, you're going to find out pretty quickly. Because it's rapidly fatal. That's why when he tells me this, I start to cry. My horrible bad luck was my miraculous good fortune. I got the cancer that was intriguing to a bunch of geniuses, and I got it at exactly the right time.

That night Jeff and I are in the kitchen making dinner and talking stealthily about the upcoming holiday and what the Easter Bunny still needs to buy for the children's baskets, when Bea walks in crying. "What is it, baby?" Jeff asks.

The girls know I had my scans today, and I told them everything was clear. But I can understand they might need their mom to say it a few more times.

"Please don't whisper," she pleads. "It makes me think Mommy has cancer again. You two whisper when Mama has cancer. I used to think," she adds, "whenever I heard you and Daddy going *hiss hiss*

hiss in the other room it meant that you must be planning a surprise for us. I didn't know you could be talking about something bad. But now I know."

"Yeah, guys," Lucy hollers in from the living room. "When your mom's had cancer twice it's not that fun to hear your parents being all secretive in the other room." Lately she will randomly ask me how my day was, and when I say, "Fine," she'll press the question further. "Are you really fine? Is everything okay? You promise you'll tell me if something is wrong?" she asks, and I tell her yes to everything and tell her again when she asks again.

Lucy comes in to the kitchen now and puts her arms around me. She is teary-eyed. "Last week after Gilda's, I was going to bed and it hit me how serious this was. Other people's parents are really sick, and I started to realize what could have happened to you and got scared." I look at Bea's eight-year-old face, still so full of trust, and Lucy's, so full of worry. We all lose innocence along the way. We all learn that not all surprises are happy ones. But I wish my babies had been able to believe it just a little longer.

CHAPTER 20

It's Not a Sprint

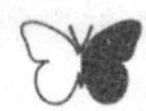

August 2012

The subway car is jam-packed, and at least one person on it has not showered in recent memory. Outside, it's a lovely summer day, but I'm off to spend it in treatment. Normally I prefer to do treatment days alone. They are long and often tedious, and I like to spend them reading and watching movies and not having to make conversation in between the blood draws and having drugs shot into my veins. But now, Jeff has taken a day off from work to come along with me today to meet my medical team (and, I imagine, get in on the free Shasta). He wants to see for himself what my experience is.

Refreshingly, unlike last summer and the summer before, I don't have cancer. In honor of that achievement, I'm lately training for the New York City Marathon, as a fundraising effort with the Gilda's Club team. My first marathon would have been a physical challenge even if I hadn't been in a clinical trial, but training through the swampy city summer has been hard-core, especially the treatment weeks, when the drugs wipe me out. I've had some bronchial issues and shortness of breath, so I have had to accept that I won't finish the race quickly. Doing it at all is what's important. I need to be something other than that patient in that clinical trial. I need to prove to myself that I can be something after disease I hadn't been before it. I'm six months cancer free, and I'm trying to figure out who I am these days. Trying to understand all the surprisingly new baggage that my cancer still brings to me, even after it's ostensibly gone.

I've lived a relatively risk-averse life, but sometimes, I have waves of panic, an almost religious fear that if I had just worn more sunscreen or not eaten sugar or been a more positive person, I wouldn't have found myself in this jam.

Even though I know, intellectually, my cancer didn't necessarily care how virtuously I've lived, I cannot shake this strange sense of shame associated with my disease. I have to fight a sense of failure, like being alabaster skinned and getting sunburns as a child was my fault, or that my cancer was a manifestation of my unresolved emotional issues. I have to work at not blaming myself for what I've been through. It's not always easy when the first thing people inevitably ask when you tell them you've had melanoma is "Did you tan?" No, I didn't. But would I not deserve my clinical trial, my miraculous healing, if I had? I've read articles that describe melanoma as a "lifestyle choice" disease. A few nights ago, at a boring party full of low-tier media types like myself to celebrate the release of, I don't know, something that meant free mini-quiches for showing up, I ran into a woo-woo, New Agey acquaintance who, in a very misguided attempt at party small talk, asked me, "Don't you think it's telling that you got cancer on your head? I mean, you are a person who spends a lot of time in her thoughts, right?"

Here's a science lesson: UV rays from the sun activate the melanin in the body. When a person is standing or sitting upright out of doors, the first place the sun's rays hit is the top of the head. Those of northern European ancestry and pale complexion are more vulnerable to the effects. But sure, I thought my way into that.

I cannot imagine how much harder it must be for people with conditions even more closely associated with behavior, the stigma they have to deal with for being unfortunate enough to get lung cancer or emphysema or HIV. I have had three family members die of smoking-related diseases, and I can attest that they were human beings who didn't deserve to suffer either. And I have learned that all the weirdness cancer brings isn't reserved just for the person who had it.

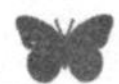

"I don't understand," Jeff says as the rush hour A train thunders toward Columbus Circle. "Everything is great. You had your latest scans two days ago and they were totally clear. Your treatment has been going fine. I know you're okay, but," and he looks so dejected and beaten down my heart cracks, "I'm so edgy and emotional lately. I feel really scared and sad all the time." Dad has been dead over a year, and yet just this week Jeff texted me that he'd found himself unexpectedly sobbing about his father at work. He had told me, "A locked office door is a good thing today."

"Well, you still are on the way to watch me get about two dozen vials of blood taken out of my body and a non–FDA-approved drug combination put into it," I say, "so let's not underestimate that. You do know why it's called post-traumatic stress, right? It's because it happens after the trauma."

There's this inane prevailing notion that grief only takes a year and then you move on, like it's something you can set a timer to. There's this idea that getting a clear diagnosis is a happy ending. Yes, grief does subside, and a complete response is better than dying of cancer, but it's not quite that simple. There is a whole lot of emotional walloping along the way, and it is real and largely unavoidable and emotionally exhausting.

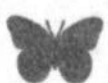

I am now in my seersucker robe, and Jeff is this time sitting with me. Before long, Karen comes into the exam room with her checklist of side effects to ask how I'm doing.

"Uhhh, great?" I reply, hesitantly. "You guys tell me I'm doing great. How are the other people in the trial doing?"

"We're still pleased with the results," she answers. "I guess you were meant to be here."

I know she means I was lucky—and I was. But I've spent so much time trying to make sense of all of this, to find the meaning and the grace, that I have to ask myself, Who the hell is meant to get cancer? And who is meant to be saved from it? Was Dad meant to? Was Debbie? Was Cassandra meant to die before her sons could even rack up a childhood's worth of memories of her? I cannot find meaning or sense in any of it, and I never, ever will. I don't know why I was brought here, or what in this world is meant to be. I only know that here I am, one of an elite group that science will someday note the drugs worked on.

Jeff and I go into my regular suite with its reclining chair and its green, leafy potted plants and its view of the office building and its bored-looking workers right across the street. I settle into my chair and instinctively roll up my sleeve as the nurse comes in with the blood pressure monitor and the IV tower. It's all still relatively unknown territory for Jeff. Welcome to my world, dear. When it's all over, he takes me out to P. J. Clarke's for a burger dinner, and he tells me, "Thank you for not dying." Believe me, it was my pleasure.

A few days later, while the girls are at their day camp, I head to the Indian Road Café in the late afternoon to work on a freelance project. I go for the coffee and the all-too-welcome change of scenery from the four walls of our apartment. Yet when I walk in, I happily accept immediately I'm not going to get a lot accomplished today. Because Leo is back.

Leo is the last guy you'd have figured to wind up sick. For starters, he's the unofficial mayor of the neighborhood. On Saturdays, you can find him at the farmers market on Isham Street, selling his art and his T-shirts. On weekday mornings he's in Inwood Park, running or meditating on a bench. In the afternoons he's working and socializing here at the café. He's a vegan. He's got a bike club. His online bio is "friend to all." He was diagnosed with acute myeloid leukemia last month.

The news of Leo's illness immediately shook our little community like an earthquake. That man is as much of a fixture in the landscape here as graffiti murals and the giant plastic chicken on the roof of the Fine Fare—and nothing bad could ever happen to any of them, right? He's always had the appearance of being strong and healthy—the guy you could pick out in the crowd by the sound of his laugh and the gaggle of friends surrounding him. The only real strike against him—and it's a doozy—is that he doesn't have insurance. Maybe if he did, he'd have gone to see a doctor sooner. Then again, maybe it wouldn't have changed the diagnosis at all. All that matters right now is that so cherished in our neighborhood is Leo that his crowdfunding effort to pay his hospital bills quickly netted over $25,000. If you get sick and you're not fortunate enough to have insurance, I suggest as a Plan B to be very, very well loved. If Leo had needed a treatment like Yervoy—which costs a fortune if you're not in a Bristol-Myers Squibb drug-combination clinical trial like me—I don't know how he could have done it. This is a fact both outrageous and cruel.

Yet here Leo is now, at his usual perch—back home after several weeks in the hospital undergoing aggressive chemo, a memorable place to have passed his 40th birthday, to be sure. He looks great—a lot better than he was earlier this year when the disease was taking hold. He's still clearly weakened, though, and he looks melancholy too. He hugs me enthusiastically when I walk in.

"Welcome back," I say. "Inwood missed you. It must be good to be back."

He smiles a little ruefully.

"Yeah," he says. "But you know how it is. For six weeks all I wanted to do was come home. Then on my first night back, I woke up in the middle of the night in a panic, reaching for the rails on a hospital bed and wondering where they were. My own bed doesn't feel like my bed anymore." He starts to sob. "I can't even explain it to most people. Everything is different, and I'm just trying to stay alive for my daughter."

"I know," I say as I put my arms around him. "I know." We stay like that for what feels like a long time, wordless and sad. People talk about getting "back to normal." You never go back to normal. The person you were before is gone. You just go on in a new place.

I will see Leo many more times over the days and weeks that follow. I will see him sitting in the park and reading at the café. I will follow his Instagram and see his photos of his raw, vegan treats and his triumphant face after his runs and bike rides, and then the images from his chemo treatments after his relapse. In one of them he writes, "When one no longer fears death and instead makes it a friend, one can truly begin living." I will see him at the farmers market, right after Christmas. "My doctor says my white count is too low," he'll say. "He tells me I only have a few weeks, and that

I have to do another round of chemo. I tell him, I'm not hearing that." He will look gorgeous, that last time I see him, when I wish him a happy new year. He will live the first two weeks of it before he dies at his home, surrounded by loved ones. And I will feel him at my back, even now, on my morning runs through our park, pushing me forward.

CHAPTER 21

The Veteran

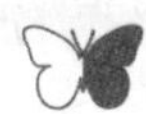

November 18, 2012

It's not the running that's the hardest part. It's how you feel when you stop.

I'm doing remarkably well. My doctors are currently writing about my trial to publish their results in the *New England Journal of Medicine* this coming spring—just in time to present them at the American Society of Clinical Oncology's annual conference in May. Dr. Wolchok tells me that our trial—and in particular, results like mine—have created a stir in the medical community. I, meanwhile, have spent the past months diligently teaching my feet the route of the New York City Marathon, with measured runs through all five boroughs. I had pictured crossing a finish line—a real, physical one—so differently. I thought my big moment would have been in my own city. I thought my family would be there to hug me at the end. But Hurricane Sandy changed the plan. Our Gilda's Club team wound up instead spending marathon day pitching in on Staten Island.

And then this morning, less than three weeks after the storm, I ran the Philadelphia Marathon instead. The experience was beautiful and bittersweet, with throngs of well-wishers cheering on runners like me, who charged from the Art Museum to Fairmount Park and into Manayunk and back, in shirts declaring we were refugees from the New York City Marathon that didn't happen. I felt loved every step of the way. But work and school meant that Jeff and the kids had to stay back at home. I have luckily snagged a place to crash, staying at the house of an out-of-town friend. But I'm in relative solitude here.

Debbie had hoped to be encouraging me from the sidelines. Instead, today she's too sick to attend. She spent the past year on Abraxane, a "good year," as she calls it. We'd seen each other most recently just a few months ago, during a relaxed family weekend together in Philly. Just a short time ago, her CA 125 numbers had been great. Under 35 is normal. She was at 16.

"I was going to be done, just one more scan," she'd said when I got the call.

As I stand in the shower feeling blisters blooming around my toes, some of which no longer have nails on them, I think how different everything is now from when I signed up with the Gilda's Club team just six months ago in May. This marathon—I'd thought I had to prove something to myself. Instead, it wound up being a gesture of devotion for a friend.

A few weeks ago they found a 2.5-centimeter mass on Deb's hysterectomy site. She's started a new treatment in a promising clinical trial of her own—she's getting a combination of alisertib and paclitaxel. And while I was devouring a pretzel at the Reading Terminal Market yesterday, she had called to say she couldn't come to see the race. She had calmly explained that she was in agony because the new drugs were making her mouth unbearably sore, and none of her doctors were around on the weekend. She was so worn out from pain she could barely speak. But she called anyway because, that's Debbie.

So this morning I'd gotten up at four and gone down to the art museum. I'd run 26.2 miles around our old haunts, past bars she and Jill and I used to stumble out of when we were roommates together at Temple that are now Starbucks, through Fairmount Park and up into Manayunk and back to Logan Circle. As I crossed the finish line, Kate Bush's "Running Up That Hill" was playing. I got a shiny finisher's medal placed around my neck, and tomorrow I will put it in the mail for Debbie. It will not cure her cancer. It will not fix anything. It will only tell her that I love her.

CHAPTER 22

Truly Remarkable

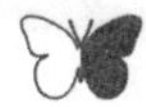

May 17, 2013

I have just made the greatest published appearance of my life. I've been a writer for more than 20 years. I've had my byline in a lot of places, but nothing compares in excitement with this venue—and it never mentions my name. I'm just a dot. I'm just a line. A year and a half into my trial, I'm a marker of something incredible.

This week, Dr. Wolchok and my immunology team have presented the results of our trial at the American Society of Clinical Oncology's annual meeting, in advance of publishing them in the *New England Journal of Medicine*. Suddenly, my little trial is big news. In a statement, American Society of Clinical Oncology president Dr. Sandra Swain says of the findings, "This is truly remarkable. This kind of response has not been seen with immunotherapy before." I write about it for Salon; I appear on *NBC Nightly News* to talk about my experience. I now learn my second drug has a cute new name that I'm unsure how to pronounce: nivolumab. It's a surreal time.

I'm not usually one to snuggle up with a copy of the *New England Journal of Medicine*, but in this case, it makes for a mighty satisfying read. "A total of 16 patients had tumor reduction of 80 percent or more at 12 weeks, including 5 with a complete response." Complete response, that's me. My favorite bit is the part that reads, "Rapid and deep responses occurred in a substantial proportion of treated patients . . . including some patients who had had extensive and bulky tumors. Particularly striking was the observation that across the concurrent-regimen cohorts, 31 percent of the patients with a response that could be evaluated had tumor regression of 80 percent or more by week 12." I am also psyched to see that "No treatment-related deaths were reported." And, confirming that two is often better than one, the report notes the "combined blockade of PD-1 and CTLA-4 achieved more pronounced antitumor activity than blockade of either pathway alone."

When I next go back to Memorial for another round of blood work in June, a new nurse tells me, "I've read about your trial. That's so wonderful." Then she adds, clearly quite moved, "You know, in Phase 1s, we usually expect a lot of losses."

I do know, sort of. I know in the abstract way that I couldn't really get my head around when I was in the thick of it. I know it from the casual way one of the residents on my trial now mentions to me how, "In Phase 1, it's mostly just testing for safety." Of course, the doctors and the researchers and the pharmaceutical companies hope that it'll work and that we'll live. It's just that, historically, it hasn't always worked out so successfully. Not in the early trials anyway.

I also know that, even with a success that is making headlines, not everyone in my trial has had reason to celebrate. The report makes that part clear too. There have been days when my team has come into my exam room, jubilant at how well I'm doing. But I know they have walked into very different rooms too, with different news, and that there have been very different outcomes for others. I don't believe that anybody ever loses a battle when it comes to cancer, but not everybody responds to treatment either. And I have insane amounts of respect for what it takes to steer people through all of it, in all its variations.

When I ask her how she deals with working in a field that's so rife with loss, Karen doesn't offer clinical reserve. Instead she admits, frankly, "It's devastating for us. What we try to do is give all the patients some level of hope, and becoming that hope is what I do. I try to mirror that hope for them, and keep myself focused on the fact that we're saving a lot of lives. Unfortunately we're not going to save all of them. We have to just be strong for them, be confident for them, no matter which situation we're faced with. But it's very hard, because these patients do become very close to us, and it's devastating when it doesn't go right."

I understand that devastation, in no small part because of Debbie. She was kicked out of her clinical trial this winter. Right around Valentine's Day, she went in for her treatment, and they instead dropped the bombshell that it wasn't working and that they were moving her to a different protocol. They told her she had a tumor that had grown to 3.5 centimeters, that they had to come up with a whole new treatment plan for her.

By the time of her latest surgery, a few weeks ago, the tumor had grown to five centimeters. Her cancer is ferocious and tenacious. She told me beforehand that they were taking out six inches of her bowels, and then, as she put it, "They're putting a 29-millimeter ring in me, so I can only poop as big as the ring, I guess. I looked at it and said, 'Do you have a bigger one?' "

The entire course of our relationship, we've been on similar paths. Now our paths are diverging drastically, and in the worst possible way.

CHAPTER 23

Where Do We Go From Here?

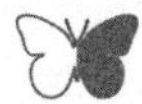

August 2013

It is an oppressively hot afternoon. Mike and Deb are in town for a quick overnight getaway while their kids are away with friends, and I am free because I had a morning of blood work and scans at Sloan Kettering. Happy third cancer diagnosis birthday to me.

We have travel tales to exchange this afternoon. Mike and Debbie just got back from a big family trip to Northern California, where they showed the kids redwoods and Yosemite and cable cars. I recently got back from San Francisco myself. I was there for a memorial.

On July 5, I had awakened in the morning and read my friend J. P.'s series of Fourth of July tweets about watching the parade and listening to New Order with his friends. That was the morning his sister Nell called to say that J. P. had gone to bed that night and never awakened.

"They think it was his heart," she'd said. His memorial had been as lively and gregarious as he had been, with plenty of vodka and much dancing to the Spice Girls.

The day outside is sweltering, but it's cool and dark in the Upper East Side pub that Mike and Deb and I are taking refuge in. We order a few plates of fries and a pitcher of beer. I keep my phone in plain view, as I always do on scans day, periodically checking. What if, after all, I don't hear its ring? What if it vibrates and I don't feel it? How will I know if there's something wrong?

For the past few months, Mike and Deb have been trying to get Debbie into another clinical trial, or even another facility that might offer a more hopeful course of treatment. So far it's been a frustrating litany of rejections. "One place wasn't taking any ob-gyn patients at all because two docs were on maternity leave," Debbie says. The secret to cancer, like comedy, is timing.

Since the news of my trial's success has gone wide, my ipi and nivo drug combination has gone into new clinical trials for a variety of other cancers—including ovarian. I had asked my trial doctor Evelyn, who's now working on the ovarian clinical trial, to talk to Debbie a few weeks ago. But that trial isn't recruiting any more patients right now, so my wonder drugs are currently out of Debbie's reach. We're hoping she can at least get wait-listed. Deb also tried to get into a trial for a new kind of chemo called birinapant through the National Institutes of Health. "I worked on it for months with my doctors," she says, "then I got a letter saying that based on my scans I didn't qualify." A few weeks ago she met with someone at the Fox Chase Cancer Center in Philadelphia about trials and second opinions, but the doctor there recommended the same protocol Debbie's current hospital is giving her.

This is the cruel reality of successful cancer treatment. You want so much for everybody to get what you got, and for it to work like it did on you, but that's not how it happens. Instead, getting better often feels as random as getting sick was. Right now in Colorado, a 40-year-old father of three with Stage 4 melanoma is in the midst of a desperate public campaign to pressure Merck and Bristol-Myers Squibb to grant him compassionate access to an immunotherapy trial like mine. He will die in three months.

"So how was Cali?" I ask Deb as we dip our fries into pools of ketchup.

"It was fun," she replies. "Everybody got along for almost the whole time." This, when you travel with kids and are confined together for two weeks without the usual helpfully distracting buffers of your day-to-day social circle, is a major achievement. "How was it for you?" she asks.

"Great," I tell her, truthfully. "I saw a lot of friends I hadn't seen in a really long time. The DJ was fabulous. Best playlist ever."

"Hey, I have a memorial playlist," she says.

"Me too," I tell her. "I call it 'The Fun in Funeral.' I have big plans for my big day. 'Time After Time' is my ultimate funeral jam. I also have 'Jump' by Van Halen. 'There Is a Light That Never Goes Out.' 'Love Train.' Oh and most definitely 'O-o-h Child' by the Five Stair-steps. What's on yours?"

"Dammit," Debbie says, "'O-o-h Child' is on mine. Okay, who-ever goes first gets dibs."

"That's not funny," says Mike. We both look up from our fries, thrown for a moment by the interruption.

"We're just kidding around," I tell him, but I feel ashamed and contrite.

"Well don't," he says. "Don't say stuff like that. It's not a joke."

Debbie and I have done little else our entire relationship but joke. Even more ever since this whole fiasco began. We have joked about our internal organs falling out and infections and oozing scars and invasive procedures and awkward hair loss and awkward sex. We have joked about constipation. And diarrhea, too, because we don't like to play gastrointestinal favorites. I almost don't know if I know how to have a conversation with her that isn't a joking one.

"I'm sorry," I say. "It's not." I imagine this is all a lot less hilarious when you're the one designated to be left behind.

I come home that evening and find Jeff splayed on the bed, watching the ceiling fan whir above him. "How were your scans? How are Mike and Deb?" he asks.

"Everything is fine," I say. "Also kinda shitty. It's so not fair. It's all not fair."

I feel his fingers brush against mine as outside the day turns into night. "I'm glad I didn't lose you," he says.

"I'm glad I didn't lose you too," I reply.

CHAPTER 24

The Graduate

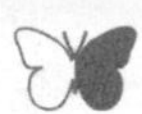

November 6, 2013

I still think a lot about what my friend King said back when I was first diagnosed. The answer to "Why?" is "Because," and the answer to "Why me?" is "Why not me?" Yet although that's philosophically satisfying enough for me, it's not quite sufficient to cancer researchers. When immunotherapy works, it seems to work like gangbusters. But it still doesn't work on a lot of people. When I randomly met an oncologist from Sloan Kettering while sitting by a lake in Wellfleet this past summer, she knew who I was, but not by name. And she asked me, "It's still such a small number of successes. The question is, why you?"

Jill O'Donnell-Tormey of the Cancer Research Institute surmises that after decades spent trying to understand the intricacies of the immune system and developing treatments that work on a sizable enough population, this is the next big puzzle to solve. "We're in a place we've never been before," she says. "We now have patients for whom immunotherapy works, and patients for whom it doesn't. We now have a way to interrogate that. Is there a genetic difference in these patients? Is their immune system different? Are their tumors different? It's unprecedented for immunologists to be asking these questions, and that's really going to lead to new things," she observes. But, she adds, "Even though people hear these great stories, immunotherapy is not an option for every single type of cancer. That's why we have to do more research. We don't have all the answers yet." The story for scientists is getting really interesting now. But for me, it's winding down.

After two years in this trial, I had a very romantic idea of how my last day of treatment—which falls conveniently right before my birthday—was going to go. I was going to kick back in my suite and watch movies all day. I was going to tearfully hug my doctors and nurses, and they were going to thank me for being such a great patient, and they were going to get misty-eyed too. I was going to finish up at my usual time, around 5:30 or so, and walk 20 blocks downtown to meet Jeff for my celebratory birthday-graduation dinner at Artisanal, and we were going to eat cheese, cheese, and more cheese.

Instead, the fourth floor is packed this day, and I spend most of it in the waiting room. Sloan Kettering is cancer's hottest ticket now, evidenced by the steady stream of patients going in and out and the constant *ding* of the elevator. I have a granola bar for lunch while I wait for my blood work to come back from the lab.

Three years ago, in 2010, I was referred for an immunology consult before I even really knew what immunology was. Now I get emails from readers and friends of friends who've just been diagnosed with cancer, asking how they can have what I'm having. Unfortunately, because of the limitations of access—or, frustratingly, because of doctors who aren't keeping up with the advancements in their fields—not all of them are being accommodated. As immunology continues to make headlines, skepticism and resistance still abound, even as the demand for both approved drugs and clinical trials appears to overtake the medical community's current ability—or in some cases, inclination—to meet it.

Dr. Pete notices it too. "I sometimes feel when I come to Sloan Kettering that even we are not prepared for the surge coming at us," he says. "We're at ground zero for innovation, and are turning people away. And then I look outside, go further afield: Are we really training the next generation of doctors to handle this? We need to think of ways to increase exposure and education all around the country—particularly in places where doctors are really good at other types of treatments but maybe aren't so familiar with immunology. We need to find ways for more patients to have access to these treatments, and for more doctors to feel comfortable giving them and managing them."

He continues, "The doctors we talk to care just as much as anybody. The challenge, I imagine, for them—that I give them the most respect for—is that they have to see so many different types of diseases. They're often seeing different kinds of patients with different cancers. They're seeing breast cancer, prostate, colon, the common cancers. Immunotherapy is still not the main type of cancer treatment. I hope it becomes a bigger part of it, because we know that chemo really doesn't work for certain kinds of cancers. And I'd like to hope immunotherapy is as good for other kinds of cancers as it is for melanoma. Is the medical community really catching up? I wish it didn't take so much time—but I understand it."

There is no question that what worked so decisively for me isn't for everybody. But my deep wish is that every person diagnosed with cancer can make informed choices with a compassionate, knowledgeable medical team. Not everybody needs my treatment. What everybody does need is attention, information, and options—and care they can afford.

At five I call Jeff and tell him we might as well cancel the reservation. By the time I finish up with my final treatment, around eight, most of my regular staff has gone anyway and my big hugging moment is instead a low-key wave to the skeleton staff and janitors. It is not special or triumphant or anything that would make a great scene in a movie. There's no music, no montage at all. It is utterly banal and boring, down to the burger I grab on the way home. Except for the part where they have apparently cured me of cancer, it's about as great as a long layover. This is what miracles look like. It's not fireworks. It's waking up another day.

Exactly one week after my last treatment, I'm back for my first follow-up as a graduate. I have until now avoided letting either of the kids come with me to Memorial—not so much because I worry it will upset them, but because I prefer my solitude when I go there. It's easier when I'm not trying to entertain someone else. I like to go and read a book and simply be quiet so I can focus on the intense emotional upheaval it takes just to be there. But I am finished with my treatment—and God willing, there won't be many more chances for Lucy to hang out with my medical team. Besides, there's someone else she wants to see.

This morning I have given Lucy a day off from school, and we've gone together for my appointment. She watches me have my blood drawn and blood pressure checked and answer invasive questions about how often I poop. She also has a delightful time enjoying the unlimited tea from the beverage machine. Now we're walking over to the main hospital to see our Gilda's Club friend, Jessica.

In September, five days after her birthday, Jessica was officially rediagnosed with ovarian cancer. "It was a blow," she'd told me, "because you hope against hope that it's not happening. That maybe they're wrong."

She had told me that the first time she was diagnosed, the doctor showed her a sonogram of her tumor. "It was beating, like a heart," she'd said. "The doctor said it had its own blood supply. I thought, I am going to name it Loki, the son we never had. I didn't want to think of waging a battle with some invader. I just wanted to get Loki safely out of my body." Then the trickster returned.

Jessica had her latest surgery four days ago. She had lots of pieces of herself taken out: cervix, spleen, appendix, some lymph nodes from her groin that will leave her with mild lymphedema of the left leg, what had been left of her omentum (which covers and protects the abdomen) from her first surgery, as well as a five-inch recto-sigmoid colon resection and a diaphragm resection. You learn all kinds of new body parts when you get cancer in them. The surgeons congratulated her afterward, so that ought to be a good sign—though she will later tell me that when she looks at her surgical report, "I want to throw up. Holy fuck. I should be dead."

Now, as Lucy and I peek cautiously into her room to make sure we're not disturbing a late morning nap, Jessica looks tiny in her hospital bed and loose gown. Her cheekbones seem more prominent. "Hey," she says weakly. "Take off your coats and stay awhile." A nurse comes in with some forms for her. "Do you want a therapy dog today?" she asks, and Jessica nods. "Can I get that little guy who was here on Monday?" she asks.

"Pepper isn't here today, but I'll send you Barney," the nurse says. "Barney is a doll." Jessica's small, thin face lights up. If you want to heal a person, if you want to ease her pain and aid in her recovery, it is not just about sewing her up and handing her some meds. It's about stuff like this: the support groups and the art therapy and the dogs. It's about treating patients like they're humans.

Lucy doesn't say much as Jessica and I gab, albeit at a sleepier, more relaxed pace than usual. But my teen stays gratifyingly present nonetheless. She doesn't pull out her phone or ask, "Can we go now?"

She's watching, and learning. You don't need to do much. You just need to share the space. That's what love looks like.

"Anything we can do while we're here?" I ask. "I used to be a candy striper." I spent my high school years making beds with perfect hospital corners—a skill that has vastly deteriorated in the three intervening decades, and one I doubt Jessica has any need of right now.

"Actually, yes," she says. "You can walk me to the bathroom."

It's a grueling process. Great care must be taken as she moves out of the bed and onto her feet. We must walk slowly even though she no longer has an IV tower or tubes stuck to her.

"You've got this, sweetie," I say. "I'm going to stay right here."

She makes it inside and right in front of the toilet. I close the door almost all the way so she has privacy but I can get in there if she needs help.

"That was a lot," she says when she's finished. "My abdominal muscles started spasming in there."

"We'll just take our time," I tell her, as we inch the handful of feet between the bathroom door and the bed. She seems not just in agony but actively concerned that Lucy is witnessing this. "I know you're there," she says quietly. "I just can't turn."

"It's okay," Lucy tells her.

The distress is visible on her face, and the journey to her bed takes three times as long as the one from it. By the time she climbs back in, she's in deep need of pain relief and ringing for the nurse.

The nurse arrives quickly with some meds and helps her grind up the pills into her applesauce. When it all finally gets in, she heaves a sigh of relieved achievement.

Within minutes, she is noticeably calmer. "I was standing up in the bathroom," she says. "I was holding on to a rail and it was like, ugh. It was pain outside of my ability to do anything to contain it. I just had to wait for it to release me."

She looks down at her empty, scraped-up applesauce cup. "Dilaudid is really chalky," she observes. "Why is it, with all the best pain meds, they skimp on the coating? Is it because they think people will swallow chalk to get high, so we don't have to pay for the extra?"

"Not worth the splurge," I reply. "You get some rest now. I'm going to let you sleep." I can see the pain visibly continuing to ebb as she gives in to weary surrender. I see in Jessica the way I must have looked at various times as well. It's hard to be the patient. It's no picnic to be the one who loves the patient either.

She will later tell me she remembers nothing after she entered the bathroom. And later, when she has her last day of chemo, I'll call her to see how she's feeling. "I'm angry," she'll say. "I'm angry and I'm scared and I'm mad at myself for not just being happy and grateful." The truth is that you can be angry and scared and happy and grateful and tired and fed up at the same time. I guess that's the gift of cancer.

December 2013

One month after my last treatment, it's a good time for immunology. James Allison wins the three-million-dollar Breakthrough Prize for Life Sciences. He says that among the things he'd like to use part of the funds for is developing a biomedicine study program for high school and college students. In announcing the award, co-sponsors Anne Wojcicki and Sergey Brin of Google proclaim that "scientists should be celebrated as heroes." I couldn't agree more. Just a week later, the American Association for the Advancement of Science proclaims cancer immunology the scientific breakthrough of the year, declaring, "Clinical trials have cemented its potential in patients and swayed even the skeptics. The field hums with stories of lives extended . . . for physicians accustomed to losing every patient with advanced disease, the numbers bring a hope they couldn't have fathomed a few years ago." The results of my own trial are cited as evidence.

Yet even though my outcome has been sensational, I still sometimes wonder, like a veteran who forever has nightmares of redeployment, what further horrors could be in store. A few months ago during a treatment day, my blood work showed that the calcium level in my blood was high. Dr. Pete had told me, "It could just be a hyperparathyroidism issue. It's not uncommon." But then he'd added, "In patients who have cancer—which you don't—sometimes it means the cancer has spread into the bones." He'd sent me to a specialist and assured, "When you're looking at people as closely as we're looking at you, you're always going to find something." It had turned out there was no cause for alarm, but I will always need monitoring. There will be CT scans and MRIs and skin checks and blood work. Until I die. And nobody really knows for sure what the long-term effects of my treatment are, because so few people have ever done this particular course before I did. But I don't need to be reminded that I'm one of the fortunate ones.

For a while in my support group, there was a young mom named Daisy. Daisy had a rare form of sarcoma. She stopped coming when she got too sick. She said the travel was making her tired. She used to say that if you combined all the uncommon cancers, you'd have about a quarter of all cancers diagnosed. Hers was one of the ones they don't do much about. Only a few hundred or so people are diagnosed with it every year, and it takes a lot of money to develop drugs. Rarer cancers, with a smaller pool of patients, face the additional challenge of being harder to recruit subjects for clinical trials as well.

"I'm not unbiased," James Allison says, "but what's going to slow things up is not scientific advancements. It's going to be what it takes to get approved. With ipi, there were three objective responders in the Phase 1. You didn't need an 800-person trial. The same thing is happening now." However rare the cancer—however uniquely each different type behaves—he says, "Cancer is cancer. What is it going to take to say, 'Why do you have to do trials in every single tumor type before you approve a treatment?' There is no reason." He pauses. "Something's got to change. We know these drugs work."

CHAPTER 25

O-o-h Child

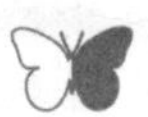

April 19, 2014

I am on the BoltBus down to Philly. I am the oldest person by decades and the only one not charging a device in the seat in front of her. I am instead staring out the window as the exits of New Jersey go by, wondering what to say when I see Debbie.

It's been a bad spring for her. It was a bad winter too. Come to think of it, the fall was pretty harrowing too. She's had multiple new problems requiring multiple hospital stays. She has trouble eating. A few weeks ago she texted Jill and me a photograph of what she fancifully described as "all the beer they had to tap from my gut." It was two liters of brown fluid.

Then in late March we got the email. "Saw the big doc today and he confirmed what we kind of knew already. Scans show tumors have gotten larger and there are new growths on the peritoneal lining. Surgery not an option. We will change chemo drug and keep doing Avastin with the hope of slowing the progression of the bad shit. Good news is we went for a nice pizza afterward and I ate two slices without my stomach rebelling."

She didn't have to say any more. Surgery not an option. Slowing the progression. She has had six different kinds of chemo, multiple surgeries. This will not be a story that has a miraculous outcome. She told me, "Our tiny brains are still trying to process, and our default coping skill seems to be dark humor. I knew when I sent out that message I'd get lots of love back, so I guess that's what we need." Then she added, "Well, that and a miracle drug for rotten lady parts." She told me not to send her any cancer presents. She just wants to be a normal person who isn't reminded that she's got no more options.

Last week Debbie was in the ER with blocked kidneys, cheerfully texting Jill and me, "No wonder I was hurting" after she got stents in both sides and a tube in her back. She had to stay a few days to stabilize. Then, because she's a badass, she and Mike and the kids went to Puerto Rico for a long weekend.

Now it's supposed to be celebration time. Jill is up from Miami for her birthday, along with Michele and their beautiful toddler daughter, Jae. We had tentatively planned to go to the Barnes Foundation in the afternoon, and then out for a birthday dinner with friends and family. We already knew it was a long shot, but then yesterday Debbie texted us that she'd been violently sick all day from the new chemo. When I get off the bus, Jill calls to say that the plans have been scaled back again.

"Deb's feeling better but she's still wiped out," she says. "She still really wants us to see the Barnes." Debbie's degree is in art. When we were in college, we'd go to museums together and she'd explain all the paintings to me. Everything I know about allegory comes from her. "Michele will take care of Jae," Jill continues, "you and I will do the Barnes, and then we'll go out to visit Debbie. I canceled the restaurant reservation and told everybody it's off. We'll just hang out."

It is a sharply beautiful morning as I walk over toward Jill and Michele's hotel. After the longest, coldest, iciest winter I can ever recall enduring, the streets of Philadelphia are a sea of trees with white buds. There is not a cloud in the sky. It's Jill's birthday party day, and when we see each other we just sadly put our arms around each other. We go the Barnes and look at incredible, deeply moving art. And then we drive out to Deb's house in Media.

When she comes out to greet us, Debbie doesn't seem weak or in pain, but she looks unmistakably fragile. There's a short crop of graying hair on her head. "I have no ass," she says. "My ass is completely gone." It's true. Her stomach is swollen somewhat—it's a relatively calm day for the ascites—but her backside is nonexistent. "It hurts when I sit down because there's nothing there," she says. "I had to order some butt padding. Then I'm going to get some fake eyelashes and hit the drag circuit."

"Are you really up for this?" I ask. She'd originally invited me to stay at her house, but now I question whether that's too much for the family. "We can hang out, then I can go back up tonight. Or I can stay in town at a hotel. It's no big deal."

"Oh, would you just shut up already?" she says, so I shut up.

Jill, Deb, and I sit outside awhile—Deb with a cushion underneath her bony ass—taking in the sunlight and talking about our kids. Then we go and nest together on the couch and watch movies like kids at a slumber party, pausing only to order Japanese food. Debbie eats a few bites of noodles and proudly declares, "Hey, I did well." The bar for victory changes, every day, when you have a cancer you're not returning from.

"Are you scared," she asks as I suck on salty edamame, "that yours will come back too?"

I shake my head. "Not much anymore," I reply truthfully. "Sometimes I think about it when my skin graft feels tender or I can't remember if I've always had some mole. But otherwise, not really."

It's now been over two years since I presented any evidence of disease. That's a big milestone, one I've been hanging on to, because a cancer researcher once told me at a fancy party that "when patients make it two years, it's usually not coming back." Dr. Wolchok has told me, "All we know is that your scans don't find any abnormalities in the areas where they were before. We don't see anything on the skin, and we don't see anything new happening. So is it possible that every last melanoma cell has been eradicated? It sure is. Can I put my hand on the Bible and say I know that? All we may have accomplished is to get your immune system to recognize the melanoma as being something dangerous and control it. You may live for another hundred years with your immune system holding back whatever melanoma cells are left in your body. And if they don't learn to do any new tricks, then so be it."

For Debbie, though, this isn't the experience. She's had nothing but recurrences; she's had one tumor so tenacious and troublesome she's nicknamed it Rasputin.

"How can you not be afraid?" she asks.

"Same way I'm not afraid of getting polio," I say. "I feel like I got the boost. I think it might really be over."

She looks at me in bogglement. She's spent the past three and a half years having cancer keep coming back. "Damn," she says. Then she adds, "One of my chemo friends died this week." She says it matter-of-factly, so I try to reply in a nonhysterical way.

"Well that stinks," I say.

"Yeah, it does," she says. "We went in for chemo together as usual on Monday, and when I went in on Wednesday, they told me she was gone. So now I don't have my little friend anymore." She reveals this information like she's saying that they ran out of Charmin at the Grand Union. I know what she's really telling me. This is how it can happen. It happened to someone she cared about and it's a loss, and it also raises the inevitable question—is this what it'll be like for me?

"What'd you do when they told you?" I ask.

"I thought, Oh shit," she replies, which is an entirely reasonable and appropriate response. "They're going to give me radiation to shrink Rasputin," she continues, quickly adding, "but it's not to try to cure me. It's just to deal with the pain and pressure."

"Does it hurt?" I ask. It's late-stage cancer. Can it not?

"It's like it's constantly pushing down on me, so yeah, I guess so," she replies, ever stoic. She's been working with the palliative care team and is noncoincidentally more relaxed sounding about her care than I've heard her in a very long time. "You tell them what's hurting and they actually listen to you and try to make it better," she says.

"Radical," I say.

The next day we go for a walk. Her whole neighborhood is nothing but pink cherry blossoms and yellow forsythia as we amble around saying hello to all the neighbors out gardening and playing with their children. "I just need to survive the school year," she says, and I cannot tell if she means that in the metaphoric or literal way.

In the late afternoon, we sit in her car at the station while we wait for my train to Philly to pull in, putting off our goodbye until the last possible moment. "Promise me," she says, "that if anybody ever says that I lost a battle, you will kick their ass."

"So hard," I say. I don't know anyone in the world who's stronger or more positive or unloser-like than Debbie. And if you think it takes guts to survive cancer, I defy you to understand how much it takes to go through it when there's nothing more to be done. "Anything else I can do in the meantime?" I ask.

"Yeah," she says. "Why don't you and Jeff come down this summer for a weekend? We'll send the kids to my parents', and we'll all stay in the city overnight. Find a nice hotel. One with a pool."

"I'd love that," I say.

Then a distant whistle tells us my train is approaching. I get to be called a survivor. She's worried she'll be considered a failure. We took care of ourselves and kept our doctor appointments. The outcomes are different anyway. That's not my victory or her defeat; that's just biology and science. And today's answer to "Why me?" is "Why not her?"

"That's my ride," I say.

"Right," she answers.

Before we had our boyfriends, before we had our marriages, before our children, Debbie and I had each other. We were going to have each other always. I get out of the car and step to the train. I find a seat near the window and hold my hand up to it. She holds up her hand in return, unmoving as the train reels me away from her.

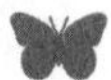

The following weekend, because life is circular, I am at a baby shower for some friends who live in a hip, quaint small town farther up along the Hudson River. They moved there for the quiet and beauty—and the proximity to West Point. Father-to-be Isaac is an Army man, a combat veteran whose stints were nearly 20 years apart, from Desert Storm and the notorious Highway to Hell to the more recent conflict in Iraq. After he came home from his second deployment, he grappled with heavy post-traumatic stress that took a long process of intense work to overcome. Isaac is courteous and smart, and when it comes to understanding what it's like to go through something unfathomable and come out grateful and deeply affected, he really gets it. I would never presume to know what Isaac's been through, but we share a respect for the toll that trauma can take.

The whole baby shower is a beautiful, joyful experience, a celebration of a long-wished-for and already deeply loved child. The bonus for me is when Isaac drives me to the station and he doesn't think I'm crazy when the act of sitting in a car and waiting for a train again so soon after seeing Debbie makes me break down.

"I feel so guilty," I say, snuffling in the parking lot. "I feel guilty that I get to go on and she doesn't. I feel guilty that her situation kicks up all of my own stuff, and then I get upset about my experience when I ought to just be upset about hers. I know she wouldn't want me to beat myself up, but I can't help it. It's all random and it's terrible and I feel like I'm doing it wrong."

He nods knowingly. "For me, warfare and combat are the worst things I've gone through," he says. "It ruins you in a lot of ways. That's the thing I didn't realize. You can't walk away without a scar. I think a lot of people don't get that. It's just whether you can see the scar. People say you look like the guy who left, but you came back different." I remember how Leo said the same thing.

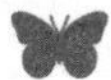

August 16, 2014

It's early morning, and Jeff and I are headed toward the BoltBus, on our way to a romantic couples getaway weekend in Philadelphia to see our dying friend.

Just as Debbie had suggested, I had booked the nice hotel with a swimming pool for two couples, knowing full well Mike and Debbie wouldn't make it. Jill and Michele are back in town too, so I'd made the dinner reservations for six at Cathy's restaurant, suspecting that we'd have to cancel. Still, it felt good to hope for a while. It felt good to arrange things and to tell Debbie things had been arranged. She was in the hospital again a few weeks ago, when the pain in her kidneys became excruciating on the drive back from their family vacation in Vermont. She was in the hospital again this week with her kidneys. She's got a little bag now.

There will be no swimming pool. There will be no dinner for six. Jill saw Debbie yesterday and says that she is considerably weaker now, and that we may get only a few minutes with her. We're coming with no expectations and no plans other than to give her whatever she needs, whatever she wants. The only thing Jeff and I know for sure is that we're going to go out to her house, and maybe we'll spend some time with her or maybe we won't be able to or maybe we have no idea how this is going to unfold at all.

Jeff and I stand together in the early morning light of the deli by the bus stop, paying for our iced coffees. "Fancy" is playing on the radio, and I consider that I am never going to hear this song again without thinking of the last time I see my friend, and how absurd and funny that is. Jeff looks at his watch and signals that we've got to get a move on. "This is going be hard and sad," he says, "but we're going to do it because that's what Debbie deserves." And because we both know it will be special and beautiful too.

Though it's only a half-mile walk from the suburban station to their house, Mike insists on picking us up at the train. "How's it going?" he asks, and we make pleasant conversation during the short ride, Mike waving at neighbors the whole way.

When we pull in to the drive, Debbie's son Adam is on the front lawn tossing around a ball with Michele, while her daughter, Jae, scampers between them. "Over here," someone calls from inside. "We're this way!" I recognize the sound of Jill's voice. We follow it over to the sunroom at the side of the house.

Debbie is sitting on the couch facing the trees. She is propped up on a multitude of cushions, her head resting against a small pillow. It's late summer, but she is wearing a sweatshirt and is covered in a blanket. Yet even under all her layers, it's clear she's all skin and bones. The soft covering of hair is still on her head, though.

Yesterday she'd been upstairs in bed when Jill and Michele had come to visit. She gets downstairs only once a day now, if that often. But she didn't like the idea of receiving guests today like a bedridden Colette. She made the effort, the long journey from her bed into the hall and down the stairs and through the living room all the way here, so she could sit with us on an August day in the sun like a normal person.

She smiles when she sees us, and I lean down to give her a gentle kiss. "Dude," I say.

"Dude," she replies.

Mike leaves the room and comes back a few minutes later bearing a pitcher of iced tea and a tray of cheese, crackers, and fruit.

"Can you make me a little plate?" Debbie asks, and he puts together a small sampling that she nibbles on slowly. Mike looks at the dainty array of foods with a gaze of mild dissatisfaction.

"Have you ever had a real Philly cheesesteak?" he asks Jeff, who shakes his head no. "I know the best place."

"Velveeta or provolone?" I ask.

Mike regards me like I'm a philistine. "Provolone," he replies, "of course," and then he and Jeff take off in the direction of Mama's in Bala Cynwyd for what I hope is some worthwhile caretaker bonding over meat and melted cheese. I'm glad they're getting that, and that Jill, Deb, and I can get some trio time. One last time.

"I can't believe our kids are starting high school in two weeks," I say to Deb. We've always been in sync; our firstborns came into the world five days apart. "You'd have liked Lucy's middle school graduation," I tell her. "They played the theme from *Star Wars*."

"When I went to Tim's," she says, "I was all ready to be emotional. I brought tissues, thinking I'd be crying because I won't be there for his high school graduation. Then I didn't and it made me mad."

"I hate getting psyched up for a good cry that doesn't happen," I say.

We spend the afternoon conversing together in much the same fashion, watching the sunlight move across Debbie and Mike's garden. At one point, Debbie's parents drop by to catch up and to show off the photo album Debbie recently made for their 50th wedding anniversary. Tim and Adam periodically pop their heads in to check on their mother and her guests. Michele and Jae run in and out between the front yard and the chicken coop in the back. The entire time is loose and unstructured and open-ended, just talking about our children and the recent Gay Games. There is nowhere else to be than right here, with each other, today.

Debbie flags only a little. Jill and I are picking up paper cups and tidying up when she says, "My cancer is acting up again. I'm so tired. It's frustrating."

"Take a little snooze," Jill says. "It's okay, we're all friends here. We're just relaxing."

"No," Debbie says, and then she says it again more firmly. "No, I'm all right."

When Jill and I return from putting things away in the kitchen, Debbie is nonetheless drowsing. But she rouses purposefully as soon as we attempt to creep quietly back into the room, refusing to miss a thing. When Mike, on the other hand, returns with Jeff from lunch, he parks beside Debbie on the couch and falls immediately, deeply asleep.

I have a photograph from the day I met Mike. I had gone over to Italy to meet up with Deb and to spend a few weeks tooling around Europe with her on our student rail cards. Debbie had been studying art in Rome, and Mike was a fellow student, getting his degree in architecture. The fall that Debbie had been abroad, she had written that she'd begun a romance with a new boy, and when I got to Italy, I was prepared to judge said new boy and his worthiness of my Debbie. By the end of my first lunch with him, I knew that he was a fittingly boisterous, uninhibited counterweight to my reserved and practical friend. What I liked most about him, however, was that he was so obviously crazy about her.

In the picture, they are on a low wall near the Vatican Museums. He is playfully kissing her neck, and she is laughing in the warm Italian light. Two kids in love. I look over at them now—she on her cushions and under her covers, he passed out next to her. Two kids in love.

"How's the radiation been going?" I ask. I remember Rasputin, the tumor that was causing particular discomfort that the doctors had been trying to shrink.

"The radiation helped me a little with the pain," she says. "It's just about giving me more time. That's what they told me, months ago. But I want to feel better. I want to get around."

Life doesn't follow a smooth, linear course. It goes forward and then back and then high and then very low. Debbie knows what is happening to her body. Yet she quite justifiably believes this doesn't have to be a straight shot into worse and worse days. She believes there can be better ones, ones with less suffering. The hope of recovery is gone, but the hope of ease and comfort is still there. There's hope for different things—but there's hope nonetheless, and it's powerful. It's not an unconditional surrender, and it sure as hell isn't losing a battle.

Her toes are stuffed into athletic socks and the rest of her feet are bare and grossly swollen, two inflated balloons punctuating her twiglike body. "Look at that," Debbie says. "I'm sorry. That's weird."

"You don't need to apologize," Jeff says. He's seen it before. He's seen it on his father.

"That's the edema," she explains.

"That's different from neuropathy, right?" I ask.

"Oh, I have neuropathy too," she replies.

"I had edema after I gave birth to both of the girls," I say, "and when I was marathon training. It's cool how you can poke the puffy parts and not even feel it."

Mike, who has been slowly rousing, leans over and prods two fingers into the top of Debbie's foot, and then traces a semicircle right below the indentations. He looks up at Debbie with satisfaction and then back at that smile on her foot that is already fading.

As the day wanes into dusk, we all recognize that it's our cue to leave and let Debbie get some rest. I stand up to go over to her to say goodbye. "Not yet," she says. "Mike, help me up."

Mike comes to her one side, and Michele takes the other to hoist her up to stand. She has neuropathy and edema and lost muscle function and a bag doing the work of her kidneys, and she weighs as much as my purse. And she is going to stand up and give Jeff, Jill, Michele, and me a hug. I put my arms around her tiny body and kiss her quickly. I'm afraid of breaking her, afraid of making her stand a moment longer than necessary and prolonging her obvious pain. But my friend and I get to hold each other and say goodbye. We get to do it on her terms. On our feet. "I love you," I say. It is one of the most singularly transcendent moments of my life. Because it's a moment shared with my Debbie. The least huggy person you'd imagine. The most generous and strong and loving.

Tonight, Jae is with Jill's parents so that Jill and Michele can go out to dinner with Jeff and me, our first double date in quite possibly ever. Debbie had advocated for Mike to join us, but he refused. As Michele drives toward the Philly skyline, Jill reaches back from the front seat of the car and we silently hold hands. I can tell what she's thinking, because I'm thinking it too. We're thinking of the little house on Naudain Street where the three of us lived in college. We're thinking of wedding days and babies and vacations and everything our trio has lived through together for so long. Of all the things yet to come.

We arrive at Le Virtù well ahead of our reservation. "Do you want to sit at the bar and have a drink," Michele asks as we walk in, "or see if they can seat us early?"

"What?" Jill replies. "I don't know. I'm in a bit of a dissociative fugue state right now." Michele tenderly guides us to an empty table.

What follows is a glorious, shell-shocked, three-hour dinner of cured meats and grilled trout and spicy broccoli rabe and granita made of orange and basil. Our pal Cathy sits down and joins us, and we all catch up and spend a very welcome amount of the time simply savoring the fleeting pleasure of one another's company.

"How was it, seeing Debbie?" Cathy asks us.

"It was a good day," Jill replies. "It felt like us."

September 2014

When I speak to Debbie lately, her voice is still strong, but her body is growing ever weaker. "I'm coming to terms with becoming increasingly incapacitated," she says to me today. She's lost most of the use of her arms and legs. Mike makes her eggs and protein drinks, and that's about all she can handle. People keep trying to bring them food, but food is really not happening at their house anymore. "It's not good," she says. "We're just trying to take it one day at a time."

She's on narcotics and she's sleeping a lot. She's bored. She tells me that they're installing a lift so she can come up and down the stairs. "Like one of those old lady things from the commercials," she explains. They got a wheelchair for her doctor visits, and a special bed. "When Mike got it," she tells me, "they said the good thing is that you can return it when you don't need it anymore. At first I thought, that's nice. Then I realized what they meant." She's nervous about her next appointment with her oncologist, not so much because of what she thinks they can possibly tell her at this point, but because she doesn't want to be admitted to the hospital again. I don't blame her a bit.

She talks about how great Mike and the boys are being. She tells me how her friends came by the other day and massaged her feet, and how nice it felt. When I ask about her folks, she says, "They're amazing. I can't imagine what they're going through." She chokes up a little before she adds, "Can we talk about something else?" We talk for a long time about all kinds of things. We talk about how the kids are settling in for the new school year, and how strange it feels for her to not be teaching. We talk about British comedies, and the joy of *Spaced*. Then at the end I tell her I'll come down to see her again in October, and she says that sounds good. I'll be down in October, of that I'm sure. But I won't see her.

It's been almost four years now, four years of Debbie's cancer. Four years of treatment and operations and emergencies and trying to come to terms with it all. It's been six months since she gave us the "surgery not an option" news. Why then am I so racked with pain and grief when, tonight, we say goodbye? Why does it hurt so much? Why is the sting of loss so shockingly unrelenting?

Maybe it's because no matter how much you think you're prepared for it, a knife in your heart is still a knife in your heart. I feel lately like I'm watching her float away on an iceberg. She's going farther and farther away, and there isn't a damn thing I can do to help. I can still talk to her, but I cannot stop what's happening to her, cannot keep her from getting smaller and smaller in the distance. I want her to not have to suffer anymore and I don't want her to leave, and those things aren't contradictions. I think she probably feels like that too. And I think that when people watch someone going through something like this and say, "I don't know how they do it," they don't understand that the answer is "Because they didn't have a choice."

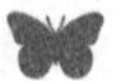

Debbie and I have a few more brief communications, mostly by text, about how she's feeling and her wheelchair rides and what TV shows she needs to binge watch, until, on a Sunday afternoon, I get a call from Jill to say that Deb has gone back into the hospital with bleeding. She had to be carried out of her home in an ambulance. "They're trying to get her released for home hospice," Jill says. She and I then have a very practical conversation about how we should proceed with scheduling and travel plans, and we cry through most of it. Afterward, I listen to "Heroes" and cry some more when Bowie sings, "We could be us, just for one day."

In an act of great mercy from the universe, Debbie is indeed sent home Sunday night so she can finish her journey where she belongs. It's just about trying to make it as peaceful and as painless as possible now.

On Wednesday evening, I get a text from Mike telling me that if I want to write Debbie a note, he'll read it aloud to her. I then compose the hardest email I've ever had to write.

In it I say, "I talked to Jill last night and we shared a lot of memories of Miami trips and Halloween parties and, of course, of wigs. You are the best fun, Debbie. You are the best, period. We are thinking of you and Mike and the boys, and of cheesesteaks, and sending you ridiculous amounts of love. I hope they're giving you lots of delicious morphine. I hit the jackpot the day I walked into that house on Naudain Street, and I've been a winner ever since. Some people get crappy roommates. I got my best friends. I love you very much. I am always here for you and the dudes. We all are." Then I close with a dick joke, because I want to end our relationship how we started it—with a total disregard for what's mature or appropriate.

Three hours later, I am in the middle of a therapeutic game of Tetris when Jill calls to tell me that she's gone. My friend Debbie died on a Wednesday night in September 2014. She was 48 years old. She died with her husband and sons nearby, telling her that they loved her and stroking her hair, with her friends sending in messages of support and strength. She died, fittingly, with the TV in the room turned on to *Survivor.*

I go into the bedroom, where Jeff is watching an old episode of *The Bob Newhart Show* with the headphones on, and stand quietly in the doorway. He looks up at me, and in that moment before I speak, a world of emotion passes between us. It's all there. It's them. It's us. It's a door closing. "It's over," I say, and I climb into the bed and he puts his arms around me. I never knew that crying yourself to sleep was a real thing until tonight.

The next morning, I tell the girls. I don't say that she passed or that she's not with us. I say that Debbie died, because there's nothing wrong with saying that death is what it is. They are both spectacularly tender and gentle with me. "I'm sorry," Bea says, and then she adds, "She's not in pain anymore."

I try to back off to give Debbie's family some space, but in the afternoon Mike calls me. When I see his name on my phone, I pick up and instinctively say, "Hey, how are you?"

"Fine," he replies dryly. "What's new?" And I laugh. Right off the bat he tells me, with the directness of an old and true friend, that he doesn't want me to send anything or do anything or make a big deal. "I just want to be as normal as possible right now," he says, and I really respect that. I tell him that I'm grateful he gave me the chance to say goodbye, and he tells me the details of the memorial service.

"I loved taking care of her," he says. He tells me how glad he was to share what he rightly calls a wonderful, colorful life with her. He tells me how just a week and a half ago, he took her out in the wheelchair and they'd gone for a walk through the neighborhood, and how "it was as close to before as we'd been." He tells me how the ambulance had to take her back to the hospital where she was born, one last time, and how as they carried her down the stairs of their house she promised Tim, "I'm coming back," and how glad they were when they let her go home. He tells me in detail every moment of the day she died and he tells me that though he's living now with half a heart, he's at peace. "You don't have to cry," he says. "It's okay, don't cry," he says as I'm blubbering my eyes out.

"You really stepped up for her," I say. "Thank you."

"No, I didn't," he answers. "I just did what needed to be done." He's right; he didn't step up. He didn't have to. He was there all along.

After Mike and I get off the phone, I pore through my box of Debbie's old letters and cards, because I've saved them all. I find the valentines signed "George Glass." And I find the birthday card she sent me last year. It has a picture of Bigfoot and one word on the front: *Believe.* I'm trying, Debbie; I really am.

When someone you loved very much leaves, you don't just lose that person. You lose that part of yourself that belonged to her. You lose all her memories of you, all her love for you. She takes that with her and you die a little bit too. That's why you have to work so much harder then at keeping that love you shared alive. You have to look at a birthday card that says "Believe," and you have to do it. You have to work so you can still feel her when she's gone.

October 5, 2014

The memorial is profoundly sad but full of the deepest sweetness and heart. Hundreds of friends and family members line around the block to say goodbye, and when they play the music mix that Jill put together—the one that starts with "O-o-h Child"—I think, Okay, Debbie, you won. One of the best gifts of the whole experience is the conversation I have with another of Deb's friends, who visited her at home right before the end. "That was the only time I ever heard her complain," she tells me. "We were sitting together and she said, 'You know what? This fucking sucks.' " It's not the sort of thing that one hears in a eulogy, but it says it all as perfectly as the last message Debbie texted me—an emoji of a turd.

On the ride home, Jeff and I listen to Jill's mix, the music of Bowie and Iggy Pop and Patti Smith. We talk about Deb and Dad and about us too.

"I keep thinking of Giuliani on 9/11," Jeff replies. "When they asked him how many casualties there would be and he said, 'More than any of us can bear.'"

"You know what?" I answer. "It fucking sucks."

CHAPTER 26

Stage 5

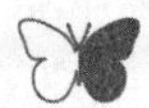

January 2015

That I am still alive remains something of a strange novelty, even now. Not so long ago, Stage 4 was the final destination on the cancer train. People like me weren't expected to get better. We weren't even expected to hold steady. We were pretty much just assumed to get worse and die. Now look at us. The 110 percenters. The ones who go all the way to 11. The growing population of a new land: Stage 5. And just to be perfectly clear on this point in case somehow you missed it—I didn't get better because I prayed correctly or because I'm strong. I got better because the science worked on me.

Talking with my researcher friend Steve is eye-opening with the distance of hindsight. "The attitude used to be, 'Maybe we can fight cancer to a tie for a while and think of it as a long-term condition,'" he says. "But I don't want patients coming in every few weeks for infusions. Now it's like, fuck it; let's just cure people. It's an exciting time, from a medical standpoint. "I've got to tell you, we were all rooting for you, but shut my mouth, how well it turned out. This doesn't just happen. The other thing—it wasn't just you."

Steve is right. My ipi/nivo combination has resulted in a two-year survival rate for 79 percent of patients—and I am happy that other trials are showing similarly hopeful results. Still, it hits me like a brick when I read a story in the *New York Times* where my own doctor, Jedd Wolchok, is quoted: "It's a completely different world for patients with metastatic melanoma to talk about the majority of patients being alive for years, rather than weeks or months."

I am now three years cancer free, one year out of treatment. What happened to me is more than just an isolated breakthrough. It was the promise of a different way of treating cancer altogether. My melanoma drug trial was so successful that in May 2013, it leaped from Phase 1 directly to Phase 3. It went from a group that started out with 53 people to one that enrolled 900 patients, all over the world, within a year.

The expected years and years of testing—and painful trial and error—that it once took to get a promising drug to patients are not necessarily the norm anymore. Dr. Wolchok says, "Our expectations are that about half the time, this treatment is going to help melanoma patients in a dramatic way—meaning significant reduction in the amount of tumor on the scans or a physical exam by the first time you look. Five years ago, we were barely used to that happening at all. Now we're actually seeing this in many Phase 1 patients. Regulatory authorities are having to take seriously large data sets from Phase 1 trials that have very compelling signals in them—and the reason is that the agents we're bringing to clinical trials have a high likelihood of working. In the past we would have some very sound scientific evidence, but we still were dealing with relatively ineffective medicines. Now we know to apply the targeted therapies only in patients who have the profile that makes it likely for success.

The spectrum from Phase 1, Phase 2, and Phase 3 is becoming much more blurry."

In December 2014, nivolumab was granted accelerated approval by the FDA under its new brand name, Opdivo, as a treatment for advanced melanoma. The drugs that I was a little lab rat for just a short time ago are now within reach of patients outside of clinical trials, which means that for a lot of people getting some really bad news from the doctor—right now, today—the odds of surviving are a lot better.

The ipi/nivo combination, meanwhile, continues to be explored for other forms of cancers. In 2012 and 2013, the first trials for lung and kidney cancer patients began. At this writing, there are patient trials using my drug combo for various forms of cancer, including lung, breast, renal, colorectal, pancreatic—and ovarian. In 2015, Opdivo was approved by the Food and Drug Administration for advanced non-small cell lung cancer. By the fall of that year, television commercials thanking "the patients and physicians who participated in the Opdivo clinical trial" began airing on television. And in October, the FDA approved the Yervoy-Opdivo combination for certain kinds of metastatic melanoma, making it "the first and only FDA approval of a regimen of two immuno-oncology agents in cancer." The *Wall Street Journal* reported at the time that the regimen "will cost more than $250,000 per patient for the first full year."

I have a lot of thoughts about the high cost of treatment, and I am not alone. In a letter "In Support of a Patient-Driven Initiative and Petition to Lower the High Price of Cancer Drugs" in the journal *Mayo Clinic Proceedings* in July 2015, more than 100 leading cancer doctors declared that the rising cost of treatment is "causing harm to patients with cancer and their families" and called for "a cancer patient–based grassroots movement that advocates against the high price of cancer drugs." Among the signers was James Allison. I agree with him wholeheartedly. Yet I also know that just to imagine a year of treatment is a luxury not everyone has. As Jedd Wolchok has noted, "When I joined the MSK faculty in 2000, the median survival for patients with advanced melanoma was seven months with the best treatment available at that time."

Meanwhile, the research goes on. There are ongoing trials using my two drugs in combinations with other forms of treatment, and more still using other immunotherapies. There are ones involving monoclonal antibodies, like mine was. There are adoptive T cell trials and vaccine trials—and many of them are seeing similarly stunning results. The field of immunotherapy continues to gain unprecedented recognition and respect. In September 2015, James Allison won the Lasker Award, one of the highest honors in scientific achievement, for clinical medical research. In announcing the award, the Lasker Foundation praised him for his work with "advanced melanoma, a disease that typically used to kill people in less than a year," saying, "His discoveries are transforming cancer treatment."

Dr. Wolchok tells me, "I feel like all those years of frustration and advocating for the religion of immunotherapy really did pay off. None of us could do this alone. I think that's really important. We needed Jim Allison and Jeff Bluestone, and we needed Lieping Chen and Gordon Freeman and Arlene Sharpe and Tasuku Honjo, who discovered PD-1. We needed all of those people to deliver the very elegant details of how the immune system turns itself on and off. And then we needed our colleagues in the pharmaceutical industry to develop medicines that could do that. And then we needed courageous investigators who believed in the science to bring it to patients. And then, most of all, we needed courageous patients."

"Courageous?" I ask him. "Or desperate?"

I know that fate will take different turns for all of us, even those of us going through very similar cancers and treatments. On a bleak, chilly morning, I am visiting Dr. Wolchok's lab to peer behind the final curtain: to see where my team has labored for years behind the scenes, unlocking mysteries inside of cells and peering into ultrasensitive microscopes. As Dr. Wolchok leads me around, I even get to meet some lab mice—the real ones—working on my trial and others. "Hey, guys," I say as I lean down toward a cage of furry creatures. "Thank you." They're giving so much, and it's not every day someone who has directly benefited from their efforts gets to meet them. I appreciate the effort, little fellas.

But though I will see some of the newest, most innovative medical equipment in the world today—and though I will meet some of the brightest and most dedicated scientists a patient could wish for—none of what I see this morning comes close to what I hear. Because today, Dr. Wolchok has had some unique business to take care of, and he wants to tell me about it. A patient of his has died.

When you work with people with advanced cancer that is often unresponsive to treatment, and you do it over years and years and years, I imagine you get pretty used to a sizable number of your patients not surviving their disease. But as Dr. Wolchok admits, "Sometimes, you have someone who's very special. This man was one of those."

Shortly before he'd died in his suburban hospital closer to his home the night before, the patient, who had been on a single immunotherapy drug, had had a practical conversation with his wife and kids about what he wanted to happen when the end came. His adult son had given Dr. Wolchok the message. "I got a call from his family when he was very ill," he says. "He wanted to give us his body." His face is a mix of emotions—sadness, gratitude, and wonder chief among them. "I said there were logistical challenges doing it from an outside hospital," he continues. "The son said, 'Tell us what those challenges are and we'll meet them.'"

So yesterday, a funeral home had brought Dr. Wolchok the shell that contained someone who had very recently been a collection of thoughts and feelings and memories. It made its way into the city in rush hour, until it arrived at Memorial Sloan Kettering Cancer Center. "He gave us everything," Wolchok tells me in awe. "There's so much we're going to be able to learn from him."

Wolchok has just lost a person who, although not a close friend or relation, was nonetheless a human being he respected and was invested in. His regard for him as a person is clear. His fascination with his body as a specimen is also evident. "The family was incredibly helpful," he says. "And we were very grateful."

I've had doctors who possess the detachment of auto mechanics—ones who, like the guy who viewed me as "the tumor," see patients solely as their individual parts. Some of them are capable and efficient healers, the kind with a robust track record of success. But when I am with Dr. Wolchok, I am aware that I have found a physician who somehow can see both the patient *and* the parts. That's how we've been able to collaborate on my care, and why I've been able to trust him so completely with it. Now, in this lab—his lab—seeing how seriously he takes that trust, even from a patient who has died, I have a newfound admiration for him. And I know beyond all doubt that cremation versus burial isn't a top consideration anymore. I've already given my blood and urine and mucus and flesh to science—but God willing, I'm not nearly done. I want to be as generous in my final act as Dr. Wolchok's newly departed patient was. I want to be able to give that gift, too: to die knowing that I can still be useful to scientists—and, I hope, ultimately, to other patients.

I am not brave. But I am proud. I'm proud to know so many of the men and women who are making medical breakthroughs possible. I'm proud to know that the cancer cells that tried to kill me are part of the research that is now being used to try to save other people. Because for the rest of my life I am going to have to comb my hair against the natural part to cover up five centimeters of bare flesh. The place where I got sick. The place where I was changed. The place where the story of Patient 1626 began. And every time I look at that ravaged head of mine, I am going to try not to just see Götterdämmerung; I am going to try to see the beginning of my little part of medical history.

February 9, 2015

I am sitting at the Indian Road Café on a winter afternoon near what would have been Debbie's birthday, listening to Lou Reed offering advice on which side to take a walk and writing these words. I am sitting with a perfect view of Leo's old perch by the door. I am sitting on the same stool I sat on when I came here the day I found out I had another malignant tumor. And I am raising a glass to all of us. I am raising a glass to something Jeff said to me recently that best sums up the last few years. "Healing isn't the same as curing, but healing is good stuff," he'd said. "Healing is fine. Let's go with that." So here's to healing. And not just with regard to the cancer.

I know people who've been through near-fatal disease are expected to become rousing exemplars of kicking ass. But cancer did a very good job of kicking mine. I'm not some TV movie, singing P!nk songs into my hairbrush and getting all wise and inspirational. Instead, a once carefree wedge of my personality is now permanently removed, replaced by a very real and often horrible sense of the fragility of life. There are days when I think I've had this monumental experience. I'm a different person. So how can I have lived through all of this and still get so pissed somebody's clipping his nails on the A train?

I fail all the time. I snap at the kids. I stay up too late. I forget to bring a cloth bag to the supermarket. I struggle with my guilt for getting sick, and my guilt for getting better. I am reminded daily that there's nothing about getting a disease that's inherently ennobling, and in real life, there's a whole lot of physical pain and emotional trauma in the mix as well. But if enduring illness and death and facing your mortality and losing people you love doesn't teach you something, you're probably a dope. So here's what it taught me. It's taught me that kale and prayer are terrific and necessary; and also that if you get cancer, you can't kale your way out of it and you can't pray your way out of it. But if you are very, very lucky, you may be able to science your way out of it. It's taught me that heartbreak and gratitude can coexist. It's taught me that the dramatic and the banal can too. It's taught me that you must accept that life isn't fair, and that randomness can work in your favor as often as it screws you. It's taught me that the gift of cancer is a terrible gift. The best you can do with it is try to make it count for something. That, as I figure it, is the work of the rest of my life. And that work will never be a battle. It will instead be what it's always been. A love story.

Want to help?

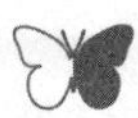

The world does not lack for organizations that help people with cancer—and their loved ones—in a variety of meaningful ways. My own experience has been most directly aided by the following. They all do incredible work.

Gilda's Club New York City: Gilda's provides free support groups, as well as classes, lectures, events, and Camp Sparkle, a free day camp for children with family members living with cancer. It would be impossible for me to overstate the impact that Gilda's community has on its members or how miraculous my family's experience with this tremendous organization has been. Along with my endless gratitude, I am giving 5 percent of the money I receive for this book to Gilda's. If you'd like to give a tax-deductible gift too, it's as easy as going to their Web site:

https://donatenow.networkforgood.org/GildasClubNYC

Or just send a check to:

Gilda's Club New York City
Development Office
195 West Houston Street
New York, NY 10014

The folks at the **Cancer Research Institute** have been carrying the torch longer than anybody. They believed in the impossible, and they have supported some of the most innovative science in the history of cancer treatment. They're also an absurdly nice group of people. You can find out more about them by going to www.cancerresearch.org.

I am extremely awed by and indebted to the good people at **Stand Up to Cancer**, whom you can help out at www.standup2cancer.org, and the **Melanoma Research Alliance**, www.curemelanoma.org.

Memorial Sloan Kettering, in addition to being on the cutting edge of research and treatment, is also the warmest, most patient-centric facility to which I have ever been. I wish every person facing cancer could have the kind of experience I've had there, of support and kindness and generosity. You can learn more about Sloan Kettering, including ways to get involved in the work that goes on there, at www.mskcc.org.

Sources

Chapter 2: Best Summer Ever

"2009 Skin Cancer Fact Sheet," American Melanoma Foundation: www.melanoma foundation.org/facts/statistics.htm.

"Global Perspectives of Contemporary Epidemiological Trends of Cutaneous Malignant Melanoma," by M.B. Lens, M. Dawes, the *British Journal of Dermatology*, 2004: www.medscape.com/viewarticle/470300_2.

"Melanoma In-Depth Report," *New York Times:* www.nytimes.com/health/guides/disease/melanoma/print.html.

"Melanoma: Statistics," American Society of Clinical Oncology, June 2014: Cancer.net: www.cancer.net/cancer-types/melanoma/statistics.

"Survival Differences Between Patients with Scalp or Neck Melanoma and Those With Melanoma of Other Sites in the Surveillance, Epidemiology, and End Results (SEER) Program," by Anne M. Lachiewicz, Marianne Berwick, Charles L. Wiggins, and Nancy E. Thomas, *JAMA Dermatology*, April 1, 2008: archderm.jamanetwork.com/article.aspx?articleid=419633.

"Sympathy for Christopher Hitchens," by Mary Elizabeth Williams, Salon.com, August 6, 2010: www.salon.com/2010/08/06/christopher_hitchens_rages_against_cancer/.

"Treatment of Metastatic Melanoma: An Overview," by Shailender Bhatia, Scott S. Tykodi, and John A. Thompson, May 2009: www.ncbi.nlm.nih.gov/pmc/articles/PMC2737459.

"What Are the Key Statistics About Melanoma Skin Cancer?" American Cancer Society: www.cancer.org/cancer/skincancer-melanoma/detailedguide/melanoma-skin-cancer-key-statistics.

Interlude: Cancer for Beginners

"Cancer—A Biological Approach," by Macfarlane Burnet, *British Medical Journal*, April 1957: www.ncbi.nlm.nih.gov/pmc/articles/PMC1973618.

"Cancer Trends Progress Report—2011–2012," National Cancer Institute: progress report.cancer.gov/highlights.

"Obama Announces $5 Billion for New Medical Research," by Deborah Charles, Reuters, September 30, 2009: www.reuters.com/article/2009/09/30/us-usa-healthcare-obama-idUSTRE58T43G20090930.

"What Is Cancer?" National Cancer Institute, February 9, 2015: www.cancer.gov/cancertopics/cancer library/what-is-cancer.

Chapter 3: Welcome to Cancer Town

"Best Hospitals for Adult Cancer," *US News & World Report:* health.usnews.com/best-hospitals/rankings/cancer.

"Memorial Sloan Kettering, About Us": www.mskcc.org/about.

Chapter 5: Don't Call Me a Survivor

"Adjuvant Interferon for Malignant Melanoma," Alberta Health Services, February 2014: www.alberta healthservices.ca/hp/if-hp-cancer-guide-cu002-adjuvant-interferon.pdf.

"Dacarbazine," American Cancer Society: http://www.nlm.nih.gov/medlineplus/druginfo/meds/a682750.html.

"Dacarbazine-Based Chemotherapy for Metastatic Melanoma: Thirty Year Experience Overview," by L. Serrone et al.: *Journal of Experimental & Clinical Cancer Research,* March 19, 2000: www.ncbi.nlm.nih.gov/pubmed/10840932.

"Depression in Hospitalized Patients With Malignant Melanoma Treated With Interferon-Alpha-2b: Primary to Induced Disorders," by R. Navinés, E. Gómez-Gil, S. Puig, I. Baeza, J. De Pablo, and R. Martin-Santos, *European Journal of Dermatology,* November–December, 2009: www.ncbi.nlm.nih.gov/pubmed/19709980.

"DTIC (Dacarbazine)," AIM at Melanoma: www.aimatmelanoma.org/melanoma-treatment-options/fda-approved-drugs-for-melanoma.

"James 'Jim' Allison and the Checkmates," *Houston Chronicle:* video.chron.com/JamesJim-Allison-and-the-Checkmates-25653176.

"Prognostic Importance of the Extent of Ulceration in Patients With Clinically Localized Cutaneous Melanoma," by F. E. In 't Hout, L. E. Haydu, R. Murali, J. J. Bonenkamp, J. F. Thompson, and R. A. Scolyer, *Annals of Surgery,* June 2012: www.ncbi.nlm.nih.gov/pubmed/22566014.

"Temozolomide No Better Than Dacarbazine in Advanced Melanoma," by Zosia Chustecka, *Medscape Medical News,* September 16, 2008: www.medscape.com/viewarticle/580568.

"Treatment of Metastatic Melanoma: An Overview," by Shailender Bhatia, Scott S. Tykodi, and John A. Thompson, *Oncology Journal,* May 12, 2009: www.ncbi.nlm.nih.gov/pmc/articles/PMC2737459.

Interlude: Immunotherapy 101

"Coley's Toxins," American Cancer Society: http://www.cancer.org/treatment/treatmentsandsideeffects/complementaryandalternativemedicine/index.

"Doctors, Patients Say 'Grey's' Cancer Story Isn't Accurate," by Liz Szabo, *USA Today,* May 18, 2009: usatoday30.usatoday.com/life/television/news/2009-05-17-greys-cancer_N.htm.

"Dr. William Coley and Tumor Regression: A Place in History or in the Future," by S. A. Hoption Cann, J. P. van Netten, and C. van Netten, *Postgraduate Medical Journal,* December 2003: www.ncbi.nlm.nih.gov/pmc/articles/PMC1742910/pdf/v079p00672.pdf.

"The Legacy of Bessie Dashiell," by Matthew Tontonoz, Cancer Research Institute, December 13, 2013: www.cancerresearch.org/news-publications/our-blog/december-2013/the-legacy-of-bessie-dashiell.

"The Toxins of William B. Coley and the Treatment of Bone and Soft-Tissue Sarcomas," by Edward F. McCarthy, *Iowa Orthopaedic Journal,* 2006: http://www.ncbi.nlm.nih.gov/pmc/articles/PMC1888599.

Chapter 9: Spring Breakdown

"A Record Year for the Pharmaceutical Lobby in '07," by M. Asif Ismail, the Center for Public Integrity, June 24, 2008: www.publicintegrity.org/2008/06/24/5779/record-year-pharmaceutical-lobby-07.

Chapter 10: Spring Breakthrough

"Approval for Drug That Treats Melanoma," by Andrew Pollack, *New York Times,* March 25, 2011: www.nytimes.com/2011/03/26/business/26drug.html.

"Cancer Treatment Survivorship Facts and Figures 2012–2013," American Cancer Society: www.cancer.org/acs/groups/content/@epidemiologysurveillance/documents/document/acspc-033876.pdf.

"FDA Approves Yervoy (Ipilimumab) for the Treatment of Patients With Newly Diagnosed or Previously-Treated Unresectable of Metastatic Melanoma, the Deadliest Form of Skin Cancer," Bristol-Myers Squibb, March 25, 2011: news.bms.com/press-release/rd-news/fda-approves-yervoy-ipilimumab-treatment-patients-newly-diagnosed-or-previousl.

"Fred Hutchinson Cancer Research Center to Lead Immunotherapy Clinical Trials Network," Cancer Immunotherapy Trials Network, April 6, 2011: citninfo.org/news/articles/hutchinson-center-immunotherapy-clinical-trials-networ.html.

"Melanoma," by Rebecca Tung and Alison Vidimos, Cleveland Clinic Center for Continuing Education: www.clevelandclinicmeded.com/medicalpubs/diseasemanagement/dermatology/cutaneous-malignant-melanoma.

"This Scientist Just Might Cure Cancer," by Todd Ackerman, *Houston Chronicle,* April 5, 2014: www.houstonchronicle.com/news/health/article/This-scientist-just-might-cure-cancer-5379769.php#/0

Chapter 12: Here It Comes Again

"Cancer Treatment Survivorship Facts and Figures 2012–2013," American Cancer Society: www.cancer.org/acs/groups/content/@epidemiologysurveillance/documents/document/acspc-033876.pdf.

"Histology and Outcomes of Newly Detected Lung Lesions in Melanoma Patients," by E. C. Smyth, M. Hsu, K. S. Panageas, and P. B. Chapman, *Annals of Oncology,* June 28, 2011: annonc.oxfordjournals.org/content/early/2011/08/04/annonc.mdr364.full.

"Lung Metastases," Medline: www.nlm.nih.gov/medlineplus/ency/article/000097.htm.

"Weddings: Jedd Wolchok and Karen Popkin," *New York Times,* October 24, 1993: www.nytimes.com/1993/10/24/style/weddings-jedd-wolchok-and-karen-popkin.html.

"What Are the Survival Rates for Melanoma Skin Cancer, by Stage?," American Cancer Society: www.cancer.org/cancer/skincancer-melanoma/detailedguide/melanoma-skin-cancer-survival-rates.

Chapter 13: The Storm

"In Good Hands: At the Worst of Times NYU Langone Provides the Best of Care," NYU Langone Medical Center News & Views, September/October 2011: http://nyulangone.org/files/publication_issues/Sept_Oct_2011_NYU_News_Views.pdf.

"MSKCC Staff Rises to the Challenge of Hurricane Irene," Memorial Sloan Kettering Cancer Center News, December 2011: www.mskcc.org/sites/www.mskcc.org/files/node/12154/image/december-2011-center-news.pdf.

Chapter 14: Stage 4

"Approval for Drug That Treats Melanoma," by Andrew Pollack, *New York Times,* March 25, 2011: www.nytimes.com/2011/03/26/business/26drug.html.

"FDA Approval for Vemurafenib," National Cancer Institute, August 17, 2011: www.cancer.gov/about-cancer/treatment/drugs/fda-vemurafenib.

"Ipilimumab," Bristol-Myers Squibb Clinical Study Report for MDX010-20: ctr.bms.com/pdf//CA184-002%20ST%20(MDX010-20).pdf.

"Melanoma," Cancer Research Institute, May 2015: www.cancerresearch.org/cancer-immunotherapy/impacting-all-cancers/melanoma.

"Study Details Adverse Events in Pivotal Ipilimumab Trial," by Ben Leach, OncLive, August 16, 2013: www.onclive.com/publications/Oncology-live/2013/July-2013/Study-Details-Adverse-Events-in-Pivotal-Ipilimumab-Trial.

"Targeting Tim-3 and PD-1 Pathways to Reverse T Cell Exhaustion and Restore Anti-Tumor Immunity," by Kaori Sakuishi, Lionel Apetoh, Jenna M. Sullivan, Bruce R. Blazar, Vijay K. Kuchrool, and Ana C. Anderson, *The Journal of Experimental Medicine,* September 6, 2010: jem.rupress.org/content/207/10/2187.long.

"Which Drug, and When, for Patients With BRAF-Mutant Melanoma?" by S. Jang and M.B. Atkins, *Lancet Oncology,* February 2013: www.ncbi.nlm.nih.gov/pubmed/23369684.

Chapter 15: Lab Rat

"Nivolumab Plus Ipilimumab in Advanced Melanoma," by Jedd D. Wolchok, Harriet Kluger, Margaret K. Callahan, Michael A. Postow, Naiyer A. Rizvi, et al., *New England Journal of Medicine,* July 11, 2013: www.nejm.org/doi/full/10.1056/NEJMoa1302369.

"Transforming Clinical Research in the United States: Challenges and Opportunities: Workshop Summary," Institute of Medicine (US) Forum on Drug Discovery, Development, and Translation, National Academies Press (US), 2010: www.ncbi.nlm.nih.gov/books/NBK50895/.

Interlude: How to Make a Drug

"A New Member of the Immunoglobulin Superfamily—CTLA-4," by J. F. Brunet, F. Denizot, M. F. Luciani, M. Roux-Dosseto, M. Suzan, M. G. Mattei, and P. Golstein, *Nature,* 1987: www.ncbi.nlm.nih.gov/pubmed/3496540.

"Bristol-Myers Buys Medarex Drugmaker for $2.4 Billion (Update3)," by Tom Randall, *Bloomberg,* July 23, 2009: www.bloomberg.com/apps/news?pid=newsarchive&sid=aZWoVAXYGSgA.

"Enhancement of Antitumor Immunity by CTLA-4 Blockade," by Dana R. Leach, Matthew F. Krummel, and James P. Allison, *Science,* March 22, 1996: www.sciencemag.org/content/271/5256/1734.short.

"Human Antibodies From Transgenic Animals," by Nils Lonberg, *Nature Biotechnology,* September 7, 2005: www.nature.com/nbt/journal/v23/n9/full/nbt1135.html.

"Monster Mice," by Stephan Herrera, *Forbes,* March 8, 1999: www.forbes.com/forbes/1999/0308/6305136a.html.

"The T-Cell Army," by Jerome Groopman, *New Yorker,* April 23, 2012: www.newyorker.com/magazine/2012/04/23/the-t-cell-army.

"Transgenic Non-Human Animals Capable of Producing Heterologous Antibodies," inventors Nils Lonberg and Robert M. Kay, November 10, 1994: www.google.com/patents/CA2161351A1?cl=en.

Chapter 16: The Trial

"Ipilimumab (Yervoy) Prolongs Survival in Advanced Melanoma," by Chris Fellner, *Pharmacy & Therapeutics,* September 2011: www.ncbi.nlm.nih.gov/pmc/articles/PMC3462607.

"Nivolumab Plus Ipilimumab in Advanced Melanoma," by Jedd D. Wolchok et al., *The New England Journal of Medicine,* July 11, 2013: www.nejm.org/doi/full/10.1056/NEJMoa1302369.

Chapter 22: Truly Remarkable

"My 'Truly Remarkable' Cancer Breakthrough," by Mary Elizabeth Williams, Salon.com, May 17, 2013: www.salon.com/2013/05/17/my_truly_remarkable_cancer_breakthrough.

"Nivolumab Plus Ipilimumab in Advanced Melanoma," by Jedd D. Wolchok et al., *The New England Journal of Medicine,* July 11, 2013: www.nejm.org/doi/full/10.1056/NEJMoa1302369.

"'Truly Remarkable' Response With Combination for Melanoma," by Nick Mulcahy, Medscape, May 15, 2013: www.medscape.com/viewarticle/804274.

Chapter 23: Where Do We Go From Here?

"Give Patients Unapproved Drugs!" by Mary Elizabeth Williams, Salon.com, September 13, 2013: www.salon.com/2013/09/13/give_patients_unapproved_drugs/.

Chapter 24: The Graduate

"The Biology of Cancer: The Epidemiology of Cancer," by Wayne W. LaMorte, Boston University School of Public Health: sphweb.bumc.bu.edu/otlt/MPH-Modules/PH/PH709_Cancer/PH709_cancer_print.html.

"Breakthrough of the Year: Cancer Immunology," by Jennifer Couzin-Frankel, *Science,* December 20, 2013: www.sciencemag.org/content/342/6165/1432.full.

"Drugs Approved for Breast Cancer," National Cancer Institute: www.cancer.gov/cancertopics/drug info/breastcancer.

"Drugs Approved for Lung Cancer," National Cancer Institute: www.cancer.gov/cancertopics/drug info/lungcancer.

"How Many Women Get Breast Cancer?" American Cancer Society, September 9, 2014: www.cancer.org/cancer/breastcancer/overviewguide/breast-cancer-overview-key-statistics.

"MD Anderson Researcher Jim Allison Wins Breakthrough Prize for His Innovative Cancer Immunology Research," MD Anderson News Release, December 13, 2013: www.mdanderson.org/newsroom/news-releases/2013/immunology-research.html.

Chapter 26: Stage 5

"Bristol-Myers Squibb Receives Approval from the U.S. Food and Drug Administration for the Opdivo (nivolumab) + Yervoy (ipilimumab) Regimen in BRAF V600 Wild-Type Unresectable or Metastatic Melanoma," Bristol-Myers Squibb: http://news.bms.com/press-release/bristol-myers-squibb-receives-approval-us-food-and-drug-administration-opdivo-nivoluma.

"FDA Approves Opdivo for Advanced Melanoma," FDA News Release, December 22, 2014: www.fda.gov/newsevents/newsroom/pressannouncements/ucm427716.htm.

"FDA Approves Bristol-Myers's Yervoy, Opdivo for Treatment of Melanoma," by Peter Loftus and Ron Winslow, *Wall Street Journal,* October 1, 2015: http://www.wsj.com/articles/fda-approves-bristol-myers-yervoy-opdivo-for-treatment-of-melanoma-1443711746.

"Immunotherapy Combination Nivolumab Plus Ipilimumab Receives FDA Approval for Metastatic Melanoma," by Christina Pernambuco-Holsten, Memorial Sloan Kettering blog, October 1, 2015: https://www.mskcc.org/blog/immunotherapy-combination-nivolumab-plus-ipilimumab-receives-fda-approval-metastatic-melanoma.

"In Support of a Patient-Driven Initiative and Petition to Lower the High Price of Cancer Drugs," *Mayo Clinic Proceedings:* http://www.mayoclinicproceedings.org/article/S0025-6196(15)00430-9/fulltext.

"Ipilimumab/Nivolumab Combination Achieves Long-Term Survival for Patients With Advanced Melanoma," by Charlotte Bath, *The ASCO Post,* June 6, 2014: www.ascopost.com/ViewNews.aspx?nid=16293.

"New System for Treating Cancer Seen as Hopeful," by Andrew Pollack, *New York Times,* June 2, 2014: www.nytimes.com/2014/06/03/business/cancer-researchers-report-longer-survival-rates-with-immunotherapy.html.

Acknowledgments

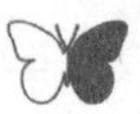

It is hard to go through cancer, and it is hard to write about cancer. But if you're going to do it, it helps to have the best people in the world to guide you through it all. Ludicrous amounts of gratitude to the following:

Thank you to my agent, David Fugate, for taking on an idea and helping turn it into a full-blown proposal.

Thank you to my editor, Hilary Black, for being perpetually smart and encouraging and full of good ideas, and to everybody at National Geographic, in particular Allyson Dickman. I could not ask for a better home for my book than the one it found with you.

Thank you to my incredible and inspiring past and present colleagues from Salon, especially Kerry Lauerman, Dave Daley, Thomas Rogers, and Sarah Hepola, for giving me a place to write about the experience while I was living it, for being so accommodating and flexible throughout my adventures in cancer treatment, and mostly for being my friends. PS: Note how I am using the serial comma here, and YOU CANNOT STOP ME.

Thank you to Dan Jones at the *New York Times*. I wish I could write a Modern Love every week; you are that great a joy to work with.

Thank you to everybody at Gilda's Club—staff, volunteers, and mostly, my fellow members—from the bottom of my heart, for giving my family and me so much support.

Thank you to the generous and passionate folks at the Cancer Research Institute, Stand Up to Cancer, and the Melanoma Research Alliance for all the amazing work you do, all the time.

Thank you to the past and present staff of Memorial Sloan Kettering, in particular the team at the Immunotherapy Clinic led by Dr. Jedd Wolchok, for being geniuses and also for being the most compassionate group of caregivers imaginable. To my doctors and nurses: That saving my life thing? Big ups.

Thank you to the friends who offered hospitality and help and humor, to my family and to me. You got us through. This means you, Carole, Carolyn, Cathy, Chez, Debbie, Denise, Fawn, Irene, Jacqui, Jeffrey, Jessica, Jill, Jilly, Joey, John, Jolie, Julie, Kristin, Larry, Laura, Lily, Linda, Mark, Michele, Mike, Rob, Rose, Shannon, Stacey, Steve, Tom, Will, Xeni, and about a hundred other people I adore.

Thanks to my mother-in-law for stepping up, big-time.

Thank you to Jeff. There's no one else I'd rather have clean my head wounds. I choo choo choose you.

And immeasurable thanks to Lucy and Beatrice, the two kindest, bravest, funniest people I've ever known. You are my role models. I love you.

About the Author

Mary Elizabeth Williams is a senior staff writer for award-winning Salon.com. The "Lab Rat" series on her clinical trial immunotherapy treatment was nominated for the 2012 Online Journalism Award for Commentary, and her essay on receiving a melanoma diagnosis is in the Harper anthology *The Moment.* She is the author of *Gimme Shelter: Ugly Houses, Cruddy Neighborhoods, Fast-Talking Brokers, and Toxic Mortgages: My Three Years Searching for the American Dream,* a starred *Booklist* selection. Williams lives in New York City with her family.

Reader Discussion Guide

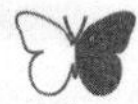

1. Mary Elizabeth's late-stage cancer prognosis was grim, and her treatment at the time had only slim odds of working. If you suddenly had to face your own mortality, how do you think you would react? What do you think you would change about your life right now?

2. In the book, Mary Elizabeth observes that "there is good in the sad stuff," and that grief is "full of extraordinary, luminous beauty too." Do you agree or disagree with her assessment? Have you ever found positive experiences within very difficult ones? Describe what it was like and how it changed your perception of them.

3. Throughout the narrative, Mary Elizabeth describes speaking openly with her daughters about her health. How do you think parents should talk to their children about serious situations? Have you ever had a crisis in which you had to figure out how much or how little to share with your family? What did you do?

4. Mary Elizabeth and Debbie have different approaches to their illnesses. Mary Elizabeth is open, writing and talking about it and joining a support group, whereas Debbie prefers to keep her status more private and her experience more intimate. Which approach resonates with you? Why?

5. In Chapter 12, Mary Elizabeth talks about how her experience has rearranged many of her friendships. Have you ever been through something that shifted what you thought about the people you knew, either because they pulled away or because they stepped up? How do outside events reveal character?

6. In Chapter 12, Mary Elizabeth talks about her ideas of prayer and grace, musing about how she separates her faith from her belief in science. Do you agree with her—and do you think the two concepts can truly coexist?

7. At the beginning of the book, Mary Elizabeth and Jeff have reconciled after a painful marital separation. Do you believe in second chances? Have you ever faced a tough choice between trying again at something and letting go? What finally tipped the balance?

8. Mary Elizabeth struggles with what she calls her "sick person's head" while observing the dramatic physical changes that cancer also brings to Debbie, Dad, and Cassandra. How does exterior appearance affect your state of mind—and wellness? Have you ever had a time when your inner and outer self seemed at odds? How did you reconcile the two?

9. Mary Elizabeth and Debbie repeatedly joke with each other as a shorthand means of coping. What roles does humor play in your life? Are there any situations—as when Mike insists, "That's not funny,"— when certain topics should be off limits?

10. Have you ever had a personal experience with cancer, either as a patient or with someone close to you? How did it change your understanding of disease and treatment? Has reading this book changed what you know about cancer? What surprised you?

11. Mary Elizabeth talks about the high cost of treatment and contrasts her own medical journey with that of Leo, who has to crowdfund his way through treatment. What do you think are the ethical responsibilities of drug companies, doctors, and researchers, and what can be done about the increasingly high costs of treatment?

12. Julie observes in Chapter 9 that "everybody, at some point, gets sick. Everybody has to go to the doctor." How do you advocate for yourself when you're in the role of the patient? What do you wish doctors understood better about the patient experience?

13. Mary Elizabeth says she staunchly rejects the word "battle" when it comes to cancer. She also grapples with words like "survivor" and "the cure." How do you feel about the words we use to talk about cancer? How does language shape our perspective?